EDDY

THE LOST YEARS

PAUL GAIT

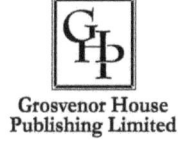

Grosvenor House
Publishing Limited

All rights reserved
Copyright © Paul Gait, 2022

The right of Paul Gait to be identified as the author of this
work has been asserted in accordance with Section 78
of the Copyright, Designs and Patents Act 1988

The book cover is copyright to Paul Gait

This book is published by
Grosvenor House Publishing Ltd
Link House
140 The Broadway, Tolworth, Surrey, KT6 7HT.
www.grosvenorhousepublishing.co.uk

This book is sold subject to the conditions that it shall not, by way of
trade or otherwise, be lent, resold, hired out or otherwise circulated
without the author's or publisher's prior consent in any form of binding or
cover other than that in which it is published and
without a similar condition including this condition being imposed
on the subsequent purchaser.

This novel is entirely a work of fiction. The names, characters and incidents
portrayed in it are the work of the author's imagination. Any resemblance to
actual persons, living or dead, events or localities is entirely coincidental.

A CIP record for this book
is available from the British Library

ISBN 978-1-83975-913-0

Dedicated

To the many, dedicated Mental Health professionals who work tirelessly and with great compassion to look after people who need understanding and tender love and care.

Preface

This novel is based upon a brief conversation that I had with a stranger on the Manly ferry in New South Wales Australia many years ago.

The man, in his mid-thirties, sat uncomfortably close to me on the boat during the sea crossing between Sydney and Manly. He was intensely polite but was clearly suffering from some form of 'mental fragility'.

In the novel I've repeated, almost verbatim, the conversation that we had during the crossing.

That man, I've called Eddy (although I don't know his real name) made me wonder about his story and I've created this novel based on our encounter, although the story is purely fictional.

Thanks

To my wife Helen, for allowing me to spend countless hours to develop yet another story.

To family and friends for continued support and encouragement.

To Janet for again spending many hours proof reading my manuscript.

Introduction

Australian Mental Health - Background

Since the 1980's the Australian mental health system has undergone a massive improvement, as community attitudes to mental health issues have changed. This then, is the landscape of this novel.

One of the key moments in Australia's history with mental health, was its deinstitutionalisation and the use of Private hospitals (licensed under Section 11 of the Mental Health Act (1958)) to supplement demand.

Subsequently a major inquiry was launched which investigated the rumours of abuse and injustices towards the patients of these institutions. The recommendations were documented in the Richmond report, which was released in 1983,

The evolution of pharmacology and other treatments, such as psychological techniques, have resulted in new treatments being made available to the public.

However, it was a struggle to find treatment professionals for those areas.

In New South Wales 'today' developments include:-

- *small community residential units to re-house residents from existing institutions.*

- *small community residential units particularly for adults unable to continue living with their families.*
- *provision of additional community based crisis teams.*
- *provision of staffing to provide adequate follow up for mentally ill people in the community.*

A number of hospitals are now however, instigating programmes which involve rehousing clients in the normal community with appropriate support services

The broad service delivery strategy adopted by the Inquiry is one involving a continuing policy of decentralization and deinstitutionalisation, based on a philosophy which emphasises early assessment and intervention,

- *that a wide range of behaviour should be tolerated within the community and not arbitrarily labelled as "mental illness".*
- *it is desirable for people to have as many opportunities for social and physical contact in the normal community environment as possible, irrespective of their level of physical, intellectual, or social functioning.*
- *further, they have a right to these opportunities.*

These opportunities are more likely than not to help them and others cope with the perceived and real problems of those who are developmentally disabled or who are psychiatrically ill

PROLOGUE

The story is set in 1980's Australia and based at a fictional mental health hospital, *'The Imagine Mental Health Institute'* located in Manly, New South Wales,

However, the origins of Eddy's fictional story go back to the recognised failings of the Australian Mental Health environment of the 1950's.

At the time, ten year old Eddy was going through significant personal traumatic issues and misdiagnosed as being mentally ill.

During the 1970's and 80's a major study was undertaken for a significant overhaul of the Australian Mental Health service, and the Richmond report was published in 1983 to identify a way ahead.

The Richmond report clearly indicated the need for additional mental health resources, which triggered a demand for more psychiatrists to achieve its deinstitutionalisation aims and the use of Private hospitals to supplement demand.

Now in his thirties Eddy is locked in to a regime from which he can't escape.

Chapter One

'Because it's your tenth birthday and you have been a good boy, we're going to buy you any toy that you want, no expense spared,' his Dad had promised.

'I want a train set Daddy; can I have a train set? Can I? Please, can I?'

'Yes of course. Let's go into town and find the best train set that money can buy,' his father said, kindly.

Eddy was so excited; He just couldn't wait. They found an amazing toy shop which had bright lights and a window display with a large train set laid out.

'Wow, look Dad! Look at the layout of that, it's so big. So many model bridges and stations and signals and look there's even several engines running round and round the track.' Eddy squealed. 'I can't wait to play with them.'

'Well we'd better go in and buy it then,' his father encouraged.

As they reached the door it opened automatically. And an electronic voice said, 'Welcome Eddy. Happy birthday.'

'Oh they know my name already,' Eddy said, skipping excitedly in to the shop, delighted at the welcome.

Music greeted them as they entered.

'That's Dean Martin singing Memories are made of this,' his Dad informed the excited little boy. 'Let's hope that they are truly memorable.

It made Eddy feel so special, he was on cloud nine.

But, as they stepped over the threshold, the door suddenly slammed shut behind them.

The song was replaced by intimidating electronic music, with a mind jarring beat. The music seemed to fill his head, the beat disorientating. Eddy was frightened.

The bright lights faded to a demonic red. The temperature dropped very quickly; he shivered in the cold.

Frightened by the sudden scary changes, Eddy reached out for his father's comforting hand.

But it wasn't there. He looked around and Dad had disappeared. He was alone. There was nobody else in the shop except him.

Frantically he called out. 'Dad, Daddy,' where are you? I'm frightened Dad. Where are you Daddy? Please come out. I'm frightened.'

But there was no response.

All the while the heavy beat of the music was getting louder and louder, hurting Eddy's ears.

Plugging his ears with his fingers, Eddy set off to find his father and wandered down a toy aisle looking for him.

'Dad, Dad. Where are you? I'm frightened. Dad.'

Unsuccessful in his search, he went down another aisle and then another and another, getting more and more frantic. Soon he realised that he was lost in a maze.

He hadn't been looking at the contents of the shelves but suddenly spotted that they were crammed with horrific, evil looking toys.

He hadn't noticed that the eyes of the toys had been watching him either, as he passed by.

Then, in a loud cacophony of noise, making piercing shrieking noises, the toys came to life. They jumped down from the shelves and in their droves started to follow him, repeating his name in an evil incantation. 'Eddy, Eddy, Eddy.'

Desperate to get away, Eddy started running. He ran faster and faster away from the baying toys. As he ran into another aisle he spotted men in white coats glowering at him. In their gnarled hands, hypodermic syringes, held like daggers. They joined the chase.

In his frantic haste, Eddy tripped over something on the floor and fell down on top of it.

To his horror, he soon realised that it was a six foot long stuffed doll. It had a flat rounded face with big saucer like eyes.

As he leaned on its stomach to get back on his feet, frighteningly the doll opened its eyes. The black pupils gazed at him and seemed to drill into his very soul.

Eddy screamed as the doll then became animated and its mouth took on an evil grin.

In panic Eddy ran desperately round the toy shop hoping to find a way out. Frantically seeking an escape he was dashing down the maze of toy filled aisles but as he passed by the toys sprang to life and leapt at him. Clawing his clothes.

With the men in white coats and the demonic toys chasing him Eddy, quickly became disorientated in the maze and ran into a blind alley. He came to a solid brick wall. He was trapped. There was no escape. Desperately he hammered on the wall as he felt the evil crowd getting closer and closer.

All the time calling for his father to help him.

Then, as if his prayer was answered, miraculously a hole appeared in the wall. Desperately he clawed at the hole and pulled more and more bricks away until it was large enough for him to crawl through.

He scrambled out over the rugged brickwork and ran away from the pursuing crowd. The further he got away from the evil toy shop, the incessant beat of the music faded out of his head, allowing him to think.

He ran into a forest. Suddenly the trees and bushes came to life and started attacking him, bending over and smothering him.

As he dodged the thrashing from the trees, he collided with a large emu. The buck emu, annoyed at being disturbed, charged him and attacked with his beak.

Eddy managed to escape it's vicious pecking by climbing on top of a crashed car and up into a tree.

Bizarrely the emu suddenly caught fire, like a legendary phoenix. The fire was intensely bright and as it died down, instead of leaving a burned out carcass, the conflagration sprayed shards of broken glass on the forest floor.

Eventually Eddy climbed down from the tree. Then to his dismay, he saw the evil crowd from the toy shop running towards him. He broke into a run and ran as fast as he could, the broken glass crunching under his feet.

But in his haste, he tripped over a bush and fell flat on his face. He had left it too late. His evil pursuers descended on him. Tugging at his prostrate body.

He felt a hand on his shoulder, shaking him. Somebody was calling his name. He dared not look. The shaking got more vigorous and the shouting louder.

Eddy woke with a jolt. He recognised the voice. It was Marilyn's.

She gazed at him; His face was covered in sweat, his hair damp from the fear. his pyjamas wet and warm. There was a smell of urine.

'Eddy have you had that nightmare again?' she shrieked.

'Oh thank god it's you Marilyn. Yes, yes it was horrible.' Eddy gasped.

'I could hear you screaming from next door.'

Then he remembered.

The frightened little boy,

With his fear filled eyes.

His skinny frame shaking,

Tears cascading down his cheeks

The fear overcoming his toilet training.

The puddle appearing at his feet.

Chapter Two

The taxi pulled up in the 'drop off' area outside the large three storey redbrick building in Hickson Road. Nearby, the traffic thundered along the elevated Cahill expressway carrying traffic to and from the Sydney Harbour bridge.

'Here you are Sir. This is Circular Quay,' the taxi driver informed his passenger.

'Thank you driver. Strange buildings for a ferry terminal,' the Englishman observed, looking around.

'That's because the buildings were originally built as warehouses for the cargo of big ships that used to use the port. But that trade stopped some time ago,' the taxi driver informed him. 'Since then, they've done a lot of rebuilding and even converted some of the warehouses to shops and apartments. You'll never believe this, but some apartments sell for nearly a million dollars, or if you prefer to rent, we're talking several hundred a week.'

'Good heavens,' the visitor remarked.

'You'll find that most big celebrations are based around here too.'

'Yes, I've seen the television coverage of the impressive fireworks display on the bridge every year. Of course Australia are normally one of the first to celebrate the arrival of the New Year.'

'Too true, all the bars and restaurants here in Circular Quay are usually rammed over Christmas and New Year. There's a fair few sore heads in the morning, I can tell ya.'

'Is it always as busy as this?' John asked, looking at the hordes of people dashing into and out of the many port entrances.

'Yes because it's a main transport hub for the Sydney Harbour Bay,' the taxi driver informed him. 'Where did you say you were going?'

'Manly. I'm starting a new job there,' John explained enthusiastically.

As a fully qualified Psychiatrist and hypnotherapist, John Masters had taken the bold step to emigrate from England after seeing a medical journal advert seeking Mental Health Professionals in Australia.

'Successful applicants would assist in the reorganisation of the Australian Mental Health system,' he recalled.

Now his mother was settled with a new partner and no relationships to tie himself down, he was looking forward to starting a new life 'down under' and forgetting the pain of the awful tragedy.

Fresh faced, tall, and good looking, he had grown a goatee beard to make himself look older than his 32 years.

In spite of the long flights from London Heathrow via Hong Kong, he was feeling good and being in Circular Quay gave him an extra buzz.

The taxi driver interrupted his thoughts. "Well if you'd prefer, I could take you all the way there, rather than messing around with a ferry,' the driver offered.

'No, it's alright thanks. I've heard such a lot about the lovely scenic ferry journey. I'm really looking forward to seeing the Sydney skyline from out on the bay.'

'Ok. I thought I'd just offer, anyway.'

'Thanks... And take me on a wild goose chase and charge me a fortune for a tour of the city, I expect,' John Masters, thought suspiciously.

'I think the ferry for Manly is either Pier two or three,' the taxi driver volunteered.

'Any idea how long it takes?'

'Well there are two ferries to choose from. It depends on which one you want to take. The Fast Ferry takes about 18 to 20 minutes. It'll cost about $10 Australian that's about £5 sterling, I think,' the taxi driver informed him. 'Whereas the other one takes about 30 to 40 minutes.'

'I think I'll take the slower one so I can spend longer enjoying the view,' the visitor said, paying the driver. 'Thanks very much.'

John picked up his two suitcases and, with a broad grin, went through the large brick archway looking for somewhere to purchase a ticket.

As he wandered into the Quays, he was taken aback by the vast size of the huge brick built structure.

After a few minutes aimlessly wandering around looking for direction signs to the ferry, he became disorientated in the large complex and decided to ask for help from a uniformed Policeman.

'Excuse me. Where do I catch the ferry to Manly?' John asked

'G'day. You must be a Yank or Canadian?' the officer observed.

'No. I'm not either and I'm surprised that my accent doesn't give it away. I'm a Brit.'

'A Brit? You got a twang to your voice like a North American,' the other suggested.

'It's probably because I come from the part of England called the West Country, I expect,' John volunteered.

'What part of London is that?'

'I come from a place called Gloucestershire. It's about a hundred miles away from London.'

'Oh is it?'

'Yes you should go there if you get to England. It's a lovely part of the country.

'I'll put that on my wish list then,' the policeman said flippantly. 'In the meantime the Manly ferry you need is Pier two for the fast one or three to catch the shuttle. It's very easy, it's just like catching a bus from a bus station. There are signs everywhere to tell you which ferry is which.'

'Thanks. Where do I get a ticket?'

'Best to buy it before you board. Then you can make sure that you're on the right ferry.'

'Thanks very much for your help.'

'No worries. Enjoy your trip.'

'Cheers.'

As John walked towards the ferry, he was surprised at the complex structure of the terminal. On 'street level' there were scores of shops, bars, cafés, and restaurants. And above the ground floor businesses the warehouses had been converted to row upon row of apartments, stacked four storeys high.

'Obviously, a trendy and much sought after waterside 'des res,' he thought. 'There must be thousands of apartments here.'

He studied a map on a large display board and could see the five fingers of the huge double sided wharves thrusting out several hundred yards into the waters of Walsh Bay.

As he walked on to pier 3, he caught sight of the iconic 3,800 foot long Sydney Harbour bridge a few hundred yards away. Despite his jet lag, the unexpected sighting gave him an adrenalin rush. It brought home the enormity of his decision to move from England, to live and work here.

He stopped and gazed at the magnificent structure with its huge central arch reaching 440 feet above the water. The memorable image made him catch his breath at being so close.

'Wow. How fantastic is that,' he smiled. 'I think I'm going to like working here.'

After a few more sightseeing moments, he collected his thoughts and walked to where he anticipated that the ferry should be docked.

He was relieved to find that it was already in.

Quickly confirming with the crewman standing by the boat that it was the correct ferry, he bought a ticket and alighted on to the large bobbing vessel.

'Which is the best side to sit to get some good pictures of the Sydney skyline?' he asked.

'I'd suggest the port side to get the Sydney Harbour bridge and starboard side to get the Opera House,' the other recommended.

'Port! Is that what us landlubbers call the left hand side?

'Looking towards the bow, yes that's right.'

'Thanks.'

John carried his suitcases on to the boat and selected a wooden bench on the port side as the crewman had suggested. He sat down on the hard wooden seat and slid the cases under it, so they were out of the way.

With a big grin on his face and bursting with excitement, he retrieved his camera from his shoulder bag and prepared to take his planned pictures. 'Ah the smell of the sea,' he thought, taking in a lungful of the salty air.

Underneath him, he could feel the vibrations of the boat's engine ticking over. The vessel was as impatient as himself to be off, tugging impatiently at its moorings, trying to break free and rush back to sea. Its bow again cutting through the aqua blue waves.

Chapter Three

Shortly after settling down on the bench, another passenger joined him and sat uncomfortably close, invading John's personal space. John moved away surreptitiously so as not to make his discomfort obvious, but the other mimicked his move and slid along towards him, maintaining the invasive closeness.

The man had a swarthy face topped by a head of wild brown hair. He was slightly overweight, his rounded stomach stretching the fabric of his grubby grey track suit top which matched his grubby grey jogging bottoms. His sockless feet were enclosed in a pair of scuffed brown sandals. There was a strong smell of carbolic soap about him.

Immediately the stranger introduced himself. 'G'day, my name's Eddy. What's yours? Eh? Eh?'

John noticed the man's bloodshot eyes. The pupils were dilated and he suspected that Eddy was on drugs. With dread, he replied.

'Ummm, it's John,' he volunteered reluctantly.

'John. What do you think it is easier to be, a doctor or Surgeon?'

Taken aback by the bizarre question, John asked him to repeat it. 'Sorry what did you say?'

'What do you think it is easier, to be a doctor or Surgeon? Eh! Eh!?'

'Oh, I don't know. They are both quite highly skilled people,' John replied awkwardly.

'Oh I wouldn't like to be a Surgeon. Having to sew all those body parts back on again,' the other said.

'Well, I don't believe that it's only about reattaching body parts. There are different types of Surgeons who do other procedures.' John replied, feeling slightly uncomfortable at the strange discussion.

Eddy did not hear John's response. He was transported into a world of his own… the man's face was familiar…it triggered off a memory from the depths of his mind…. But try as he might, he was unable to penetrate the protective barrier of drugs which was keeping that part of his brain supressed and mercifully preventing any recall of the nightmare hidden deep within his mind.

'No I wouldn't like to be a Surgeon sewing back all those body parts…would you?' Eddy repeated.

As a trained Psychiatrist, John was used to talking to people who had mental health issues and was adept at translating most of the random conversations that sometimes occurred. But his mental agility had been reduced by 'Jet lag', following his long flight. Consequently, his normal professional communication techniques were disengaged and he found himself faltering in his response. 'Well …I….' he uttered uncomfortably.

But a short blast on the ship's hooter interrupted the need for a response. And much to John's relief, the increased engine noise and splashing made further conversation difficult as the ferry at last chugged away from the quay.

However, the increase in background noise didn't put Eddy off, he just increased the volume of his voice.

'Do you think I'm too old to be a Doctor, I'm 35 ?' Eddy shouted.

'Well no, I... I even know someone who became a nurse in her 60's,' John volunteered reluctantly, not really wishing to be part of the strange conversation.

'What! At 60! She became a nurse?'

'Yes that's right. So you see, you're not too old.'

'My psychiatrist said I was too old...but you don't reckon that I'm too old?'

'Well I...obviously don't know your background,' John explained, reassured that he had correctly diagnosed the others state of mind.

'But you don't reckon that I'm too old? And the lady started at 60,' Eddy repeated.

'Yes but I...' John replied uncomfortably. I... could be wrong about her age, I would think she was a nurse before and I expect she's just resuming her previous career...after a break.'

'But he, my ...my psychiatrist said.' Eddy slammed his calf muscle against the leg of the seat in frustration. The bench juddered at the impact. 'He lied to me.'

'No he might have been thinking of your health issues...oh dear, perhaps he was thinking of your welfare...he knows more about you than I do,' John explained diplomatically.

'But you said...' Eddy stated firmly, sliding along the bench, right against John. That she wasn't too old when...'

Conscious that the skyline that he wanted to see and photograph, was slipping away, John stood up on the pitching boat.

'You'll excuse me. Must go….and take…you know…photos.' John apologised, backing away from Eddy whilst undoing the camera case.

'I'm not bothering you am I ?' Eddy stood too and touched John's arm.

'No, of course not. Well I'm sorry,' John repeated,. 'I've um…got to take some pictures now….Um, nice, to um… have talked to you…Nice views isn't it? I'm on holiday …I'll go to the other side now….'

'Cos I didn't mean to bother you…You won't make a complaint will you?...cos some people do,' Eddy continued.

'No, good heavens no. It was nice to speak to you though. You're obviously a very friendly person…I wish everybody were like you…um… polite,' John said moving away from him.

'Did I tell you I want to be a doctor?' Eddy said following John.

'Yes.'

'I didn't mean to bother you…Do I know you? Your face is familiar.'

'No, I don't think so. Anyway. No problem….best of luck with your…er …treatment…'

'But you don't think I'm too old?' Eddy persisted, churning over their conversation, as John moved away.

'No, just keep dreaming, perhaps when you're …um better…you'll make it.'

As John wandered up to the bow of the boat, relieved that Eddy had at last left him, he heard Eddy start talking to another passenger. 'What do you think it is easier to be, a Doctor or Surgeon?. Eh! Eh!?'

Despite the brief encounter with Eddy, John was exhilarated by the short trip across the bay to Manly. His smile got wider and wider as he photographed the impressive Sydney skyline with its tantalising views of the Sydney Opera house and the arches of the iconic Sydney Harbour bridge.

He mentally punched the air in a victory salute. All his Christmases had come at once. The strange encounter with Eddy already fading.

Chapter Four

'Imagine Institute, Laura speaking, how may I help?' the woman asked, answering the call on the small telephone intercom unit.

'Could I speak to Professor Phillips please?' the caller requested.

'Who shall I say is calling?' Laura asked.

'Scana Landis Pharmaceuticals.'

'Just one second caller, I'll just check if he's in his office.'

Laura operated the Professor's call key on her intercom and was answered surprisingly quickly by the Professor.

'Yes Laura.'

'Professor, it's the Pharmaceuticals Company, Scana Landis,' Laura informed the academic. 'They're on line two.'

'Oh good, I was expecting their call. Please make sure that I'm not disturbed while I'm on the call,' the Professor instructed.

'Ok.'

'By the way, you are sworn to secrecy about this call,' he directed.

'But of course. I never reveal anything that goes on here in the Institute,' she retorted defensively; feeling offended that her integrity should be questioned.

'I want you to always treat them with high priority. There is a lot on the line,' he said, getting up from his desk and closing his office door.

Still connected via the intercom, Laura heard the door close. 'That's unusual,' she thought, 'he never closes his door. It must be something important.'

'OK I'll take the call now,' he said, pushing the line two button on his phone unit.

Professor Peter Phillips, the CEO of the Imagine Mental Health Institute, was well respected in the Psychiatry world. His ground breaking research and development work into the causes and treatments of a large spectrum of mental health illnesses widely acknowledged.

As an Australian Albert Einstein look alike, his diminutive 5 foot 6 inches height belies the size of his incredible intellect. Like many geniuses, he is an intense character totally focused on his work, putting in countless hours to achieve his scientific goals.

He has little social skills and shies away from the celebrity that his success attracts, hence he relies heavily on Laura's gregarious, friendly nature.

The pair work well together, Laura's energetic 'on the go all the time' makes up for his lethargy. Her dynamism also means that she keeps her bronzed figure trim for her hobby of surfing.

As an accomplished surfer she has a lot of 'beach cred' from her fellow surfers, with whom she is friendly, but not romantically involved.

Her mass of sun bleached shoulder length blonde hair complement her pretty face with its small button nose, green penetrating eyes and full sensuous lips. Her attractive bikini clad body, understandably, attract a lot of attention from the beach boys and an element of envy from their female partners.

Slightly taller than the Professor, at 5 foot 8 inches and sensitive to the Professors height phobia, she consciously wears flat shoes whilst at work.

Although she enjoys working for the Professor, his muddled work ethic frustrates her own ordered way of working. However his intense friendly eyes normally defuses her frustrations.

Chapter Five

At the conclusion of his phone call with the pharmaceutical company, half an hour later, the Professor buzzed back through to Laura.

'Laura, I am expecting a few parcels from Scana Landis. It's a Cellphone and a pager. I'll probably need your assistance to set them up for me.'

'A Cellphone! Ok, although, I've not seen a Cellphone up close before, let alone set one up. But I'll give it a go. It's sometimes difficult to keep up with the advances in telecommunications, isn't it?'

'Yes, it's an ever changing world and hopefully I'll be contributing to it soon through my next bit of research,' the Professor said optimistically.

'What size parcels are we expecting?'

'I'm not sure. The Cellphone is about the size of a large brick. I believe it's all down to the big bulk of the battery.'

'Ok, I'll keep my eyes open for it.'

'You'll probably have to sign for it anyway,' the Professor added, as an afterthought.

'Ok.'

'From now on I'll not be making calls to Scana Landis through the switchboard,' he informed her. 'All calls incoming and outgoing will be made via the Cellphone.'

'Ok, no probs,' she confirmed. 'Strange,' she thought. 'Why all the mystery I wonder?'

'Once the project gets underway, I'll also be getting you to book some meetings in various hotels away from the Institute buildings. I'll of course need you to come and take the notes though.'

'Yes, that's fine,' she confirmed.

'But again, you will be sworn to secrecy.'

'I am always discreet with office information; I'm surprised that you even feel the need to remind me,' Laura bristled.

'Oh, please don't be offended,' the Professor said awkwardly.

'As I've worked for you for some time now, I thought that you knew me better than that,' Laura persisted.

'Well, umm, you know. I am writing a major science paper,' he stuttered. 'And I'm fearful someone else will beat me to publishing it.'

'Well you know that they won't get anything from me,' she spat.

'Yes, I know that. Sorry Laura.' he said, apologetically. 'But this is a big deal and I'm walking a tightrope with the regulators about my trial.'

'I appreciate that.'

'If the regulators hear about it and my involvement with Scana Landis, there will be unnecessary complications, that's all.

'I can imagine. But as I said, your secrets are safe with me.'

'Now I don't want you to get implicated in any of my dealings with Scania Landis.'

'Right,' she said suspiciously.

'So, in addition, you must not open any mail from them for me,' the Professor directed, thinking that the cheques to fund his work needed to be invisible to any auditors. Instead he could put them straight into his own bank account himself.

'How will I know it's from them?' she asked.

'It will be in plain envelopes.'

'Oh, that's helpful,' Laura said cynically. 'And so are many other letters that arrive here.'

'Ah yes, a very good observation. We'll get them to mark it with a special symbol for you,' he suggested.

'Dare I ask what it's all about?' she asked gingerly, expecting to be put off.

'Yes…well…umm,' the Professor hesitated, conflicted about boasting of his successful negotiations with the pharmaceutical giant or the need to maintain secrecy about his developments.

'Sorry, I shouldn't have asked,' Laura said awkwardly.

No, it's just…'

'I assume that I'll find out anyway through the meetings and it would be helpful to understand what is going on if my notes are to be of any worth,' Laura explained.

'Yes, that's a very good point,' the Professor agreed. 'Well…as you know, my long term aim is to find a single cure for ALL Mental Health issues,' the academic revealed.

'All?' Laura said in amazement.

'Yes. Can you imagine what a revelation that would be?' the Professor gushed excitedly.

'Yes, that would be wonderful,' she agreed, but thinking to herself that it was an unrealistic goal that he had set for himself.

'I am fortunate to have persuaded the Pharmaceutical company to fund my research. They can see the potential financial benefits if we can come up with the solution. Worldwide acclaim.'

'Yes I can see why they'd be interested,' Laura confirmed.

'Of course there are some minor licensing issues, the Professor revealed. 'I've 'skirted around' a few minor ones in order to move things forward and avoid being bogged down by bureaucracy.'

'Pioneering, I think it's called,' Laura volunteered. 'So what exactly does your drug do?'

'The drug seeks to repair and normalise damaged parts, by stimulating that part of the brain which I've called the 'CPU' and 'EMU'.

'CPU? EMU?' Laura puzzled. Surely they're computer terms,' she observed.

'Yes you're right. But I think it's an easy way of describing the drug, to put it simply in terms of the development in a modern car's computer electronics.

The CPU or Central Processor Unit, I think of as being like our human brain. Whereas the EMU or Engine Management Unit is the part of the brain which controls motor activities or movement along the neural pathways and receptors.

'OK,' Laura acknowledged, although already confused by his explanation.

Failing to recognise Laura's less than convincing confirmation of her understanding, the academic continued, lost in the beauty of his science. 'These receptors are more developed in some people than others and I believe that they are associated with 'Intuition', pre-cognisance and paranormal abilities.'

'Interesting,' Laura said, unconvincingly. 'And the drug does what?' she queried, trying to grapple with his explanation.

'It alters the speed at which the receptors work. The aim is to increase the speed to a near normal level,' the Professor divulged conspiratorially.

'Well, your secret's safe with me,' Laura confirmed, still baffled by his so called 'simplistic' scientific explanation and wishing to end the technical discussion.

Chapter Six

Unsure of where in Manly that he needed to get to, John got a taxi from the Manly Ferry port to his new employer at the Imagine Mental Health Institute. During the short journey John admired the neat, ordered seaside community, bustling with holidaymakers and locals which reminded him of Cornwall in the UK.

'I think I'm going to like this place,' he thought. 'I can't wait to do some sightseeing.'

After the ten minute journey, the taxi drew up outside a small office block.

'Here we are,' the taxi driver announced.

John looked at the building. It had none of the usual trappings of a hospital, apart from a small medical symbol on a plaque by the door, it could have housed any business. The four storey private mental health hospital was smaller than he was expecting.

John paid the taxi driver, picked up his two suitcases and walked up the short flight of concrete steps to the large glass entrance door.

He pushed it open and walked through the small lobby, it's highly polished floor indicating a meticulous attention to cleanliness.

A receptionist, sat at a small pine clad desk, she was dressed in a smart business suit and white blouse, her long blonde hair cascading over her shoulders. She looked up as he entered.

John was pleased with his first impression of the Institute 'This looks good,' he thought. 'Very professional looking.

'Good afternoon sir, how may I help?' Laura asked.

'Good afternoon. I've an appointment with Professor Phillips,' he told her.

'Who shall I say wants to see him?'

'Sorry, yes my name is John, John Masters, Laura,' he added, spotting her name badge. 'I've come to start my new job here.'

'Oh, that's good. I had heard that we were expecting a new Doctor. Well, welcome to the Imagine Mental Health Institute. Pleased to meet you,' she smiled extending her hand.

'Well that's a nice greeting,' he thought.

He put down his suitcases and gently shook her soft manicured hand, maintaining eye contact with her as he did so. 'Beautiful green eyes,' he thought.

'I'll just call the Professor to see if he's free and then I'll take you up to his office,' Laura informed him, reaching for her intercom, and 'buzzed' the Professor.

The Professor answered quickly.

'Yes Laura?'

'I have a Doctor Masters here at reception,' she announced.

'Excellent news. Please bring him up.'

'Ok, will do.'

Laura put her small switchboard on 'Night Service' and stood up. 'I should leave your suitcases here behind my desk. We'll come back for them later. Please follow me,' she said, heading for the lift. 'He's on the fourth floor'.

'Thanks.'

She pressed the lift button and the doors immediately opened. John invited her to go in before himself.

'Chivalry isn't dead after all,' she said, stepping in. 'Thank you kind sir.'

As she entered the lift John was able to admire her trim figure and was treated to the heady bouquet of her perfume, which made him feel suddenly self-conscious about his own body odour.

'You'll pardon me if I smell less than fresh,' he apologised. I haven't had a shower for over twenty four hours.'

'No, you're alright. I'm not overwhelmed by your BO, I don't need a clothes peg,' she joked.

'Thank goodness for that. That's one of the irritations about these long haul flights isn't it, being unable to shower.'

'Yes, you're right. Never mind, after you've seen the Professor, I'll show you to your flat so you can freshen up there,' she suggested.

'I shall look forward to it.'

'Good.'

'You know, it's awfully quiet in here,' he said, as the lift purred it's way upwards. 'It's not like most hospitals. Does the building actually have patient beds?'

'Yes, we are quite a small hospital. There are only twenty beds, ten on the ground floor and ten on the first floor. The rest of the building is used for a pharmacy, labs, offices, and staff flats. Although some of the medical staff choose to live off the premises in their own apartments nearby. Gives them a break away from the…'

'The mad house?' John interrupted. 'Oops, I suppose that's rather inappropriate,' he said realising his indiscretion.

'Probably, but you're about right. Not because of the patients, but because of the usual chaos surrounding the Institute,' Laura giggled. 'But I suggest you don't use the same terminology with the Professor.'

'Blame the Jet lag,' he apologised. 'I'm not usually that tactless.'

'We also have a number of patients living off site in the sheltered housing blocks nearby.'

'Interesting. A move away from institutionalisation then?'

'Yes, we are part of the trial to put Care into the Community and to get patients out of the various institutions,' Laura advised him.

'How's it going?'

'As far as I can gather, we have mixed results both from the patients and the community. But I'm sure the Professor will fill you in with the details.'

The lift slowed and stopped with a bump as the doors opened on to a carpeted area.

'Please follow me,' she invited, stepping out of the lift.

She led him along a short corridor to a door bearing a named plaque, *Professor Peter Phillips Chief Executive Officer.*

Chapter Seven

Laura knocked on the Professor's door and awaited the invitation to enter.

'Come in,' came the Professor's invitation.

Laura opened the door and held it open for John. In the narrow doorway he brushed against her as he entered.

The Professor stood and walked out from behind his paper strewn desk, extending his hand.

John's immediate impression was that he was an Albert Einstein look-a-like. And was sporting the signature mass of ill-disciplined white hair.

'Doctor Masters, pleased to see you,' he said smiling. 'You'll pardon the mess. I seem to work better in an environment of chaos,' he apologised, gesturing at the pandemonium of paperwork scattered around the floor.

John looked around the untidy room. Behind the Professor there were rows and rows of books standing or lying in higgledy-piggledy order on sagging bookshelves.

Amidst the paperwork 'blizzard' on his large antique oak desk, he had a high power microscope in the centre surrounded by test tubes and chemistry paraphernalia.

On the periphery of his cluttered desk a necklace of opened scientific books sprouting page markers.

Being an advocate of the concept of the 'tidy desk means tidy mind', John was appalled and wondered, 'How can anyone work effectively in such chaos?'

'Please call me John,' the newcomer invited. 'I'm still getting used to the Doctor title. I keep looking behind me to see who is being addressed,' he joked.

'John it is then. Thank you Laura. Would you mind getting us two cups of tea please?'

'No probs,' she said, leaving and gently closing the door.

'Please take a seat John. I'm so glad that you decided to join us after all.'

'Yes likewise, although the challenges of the dreaded Australian immigration points system was getting to me. However, we persisted and here I am,' John smiled.

'Have you settled in to your flat yet?'

'No not yet. I've only just arrived and left my cases in the lobby downstairs. But I won't be sorry to put my head down for a few hours. The excitement of being here is now starting to be 'ambushed' by the jet lag.'

'How was your journey?'

'Oh, The flight was long, boring and uncomfortable. No leg room. I have long legs and the airlines reduce the distance between seats and cram passengers in to maximise their profit at the same time minimising passenger comfort.'

'I sympathise. But I very rarely leave the office, let alone fly. How did you get from the airport to Manly?'

'I got a taxi from the airport to Circular Quay and came across the bay on the ferry. Actually, I met a very interesting character on the ferry, whom I suspect has mental health issues.'

'Oh, I expect that will be Eddy,' the Professor volunteered.

'Eddy! Yes I think that was his name. You're right. How did you know?'

'Oh that's one of his daily routines; he enjoys going on the ferries. Fortunately, the crews take it in good part and put up with him.'

'Doesn't he upset the passengers?'

'Yes occasionally. We do get the odd complaint. But he isn't violent, just occasionally irritating.'

'He's got a strange accent. Talks with a bit of a lisp.'

'Yes. That's his smooth tongue from the years of medication, I'm afraid. Funnily enough, you'll meet him again shortly. He will be one of your charges,' the Professor revealed.

'Really?' John said. 'Well at least I've seen him in his normal environment. And we've already done the introductions,' he chuckled.

'Eddy has been with us for some time now and appears to be enjoying his freedom from the institutions he was formerly in.'

There was a knock on the door and Laura entered with a tray and two cups of tea, a jug of milk and a bowl of sugar lumps.

'Thank you Laura,' John said smiling.

'My pleasure,' she said, heading for the door.

'Before you go Laura,' the Professor said quickly.

'Yes Professor?'

'When he's ready, would you mind showing John the local sights, so he can orientate himself around Manly.'

'I wouldn't mind, not at all. I'd be delighted in fact. But I assume John, that you are currently a bit jet lagged?' she queried. 'Do you need a few days to get your body clock working to Aussie time?'

'No, I'm all for a sight-seeing trip, if you don't mind?. So long as I can get a couple of hours sleep soon, I'll be ready. I would like to readjust to Australian time quickly anyway.'

'Ok, it's a date then.' Laura blushed, suddenly realising what she'd implied. 'Umm. Well...ahh...when you have finished with the Professor, if you'd like to come back to reception, I'll show you to your flat and we can arrange for the tour time then.'

'Thanks Laura.'

Chapter Eight

As Laura left the office the Professor sat down and picked up the milk jug. I assume that you take milk, John' he said, pausing.

'Yes, please.'

The Professor poured the milk into the cups and quickly followed with the tea pot and tea strainer.

'One of these days someone will invent a better method of brewing tea,' he said, handing John his cup.

'Yes, I've often thought that if they put tea leaves in individual porous bags that would produce much more consistent cups of tea,' John suggested.

'Yes good idea. Perhaps you ought to market it?'

'One of these days, perhaps,' John said sipping his tea.

'Anyway, I'm glad that you've joined us. We've had recruiting challenges for suitably qualified people,' the Professor explained. 'I am personally heavily involved in a special project and in desperate need of help to give me some space to run the day to day operations. So to have you on board is going to take a load off my shoulders.'

'Can't wait to start,' John said eagerly.

'Why did you decide to become a psychiatrist in the first place?' The Professor asked.

'My mother.'

'She persuaded you?'

'No. She is a delicate soul and suffers from bouts of depression, so I decided to try and do something about it.'

'So you became a psychiatrist to help your mother? That's very noble of you.'

'Yes. I did a lot of research into her problem and various 'cures' of depression and got hooked.'

'Did you sort her problem out?'

'Yes I found a new treatment. Which thankfully did the trick.'

Are you a big family?'

'No. Just Mother and me.

'But you left her at home in the UK?'

'Yes, she was fine. She's got herself a new man and remarried. I was excess baggage in their relationship. So I decided to leave them to it.'

'Well as I say, I'm pleased that you have decided to join us,' the Professor said, enthusiastically.

'I look forward to being a part of your team,' John replied. 'Especially using my hypnotherapy skills,' he added.

The Professor looked over his glasses and shuffled in his chair, clearly uncomfortable at the mention of hypnotherapy.

'Yes, well I guess, some 'out of the box' thinking to treat various patient profiles might possibly be needed, occasionally,' the academic said dismissively, emphasising the word occasionally. 'I dare say your specialist psychiatric skills will also be very useful,' the Professor hedged, stressing the word psychiatric.

'I look forward to it,' John said, enthusiastically. Although registering the others reaction to his mention of hypnotherapy.

'Although we are a private hospital, we contribute to a significant part of the New South Wales programme to deinstitutionalise the mental health organisation here,' the Professor continued.

'Yes so I've read and I look forward to helping with the challenge and changes,' John gushed.

'You might also like to know that the state is recommending we use different terminology when referring to our clients.'

'Clients?'

'Yes. No longer called patients. Those with emotional or behavioural problems are best treated as 'troubled individuals'.

'A change of categorising terminology, doesn't help the patients, sorry clients though,' John observed.

'No. But they want to get away from the old barbaric labels that have been used in the past of "mentally ill", "chronically dependent patients", "demon-possessed" or some people even call them "criminals".

References to derogatory terms like "Lunatic Asylum" and "Mad house", do not belong in our vocabulary either,' the Professor continued.

John felt embarrassed as he recalled his earlier indiscretion in the lift. 'Yes, I agree,' he said, biting his lip. 'It was a harsh way to categorise people who have mental health issues,' John said, echoing the Professors viewpoint.

'Yes, well, as you know, these clients of ours are not ill as such,' the Senior medic continued. 'Although like other people, their need for specialised medical treatment is necessary and will vary with their own particular needs and circumstances.'

'Of course. In many cases, I'm sure that the resolution should also be based on identification of root causes,' John suggested. 'And supplemented by education and mindful training, where possible, rather than relying solely on chemical treatments.'

'I hear what you say. However, medication through the use of injections and pills has always played a vital part in successful treatment regimes,' the Professor countered quickly.

'Yes, agreed. Currently they do.' John concurred. 'However treatment methods are still evolving, as you know.'

'Yes of course. I would like to think that the treatments we provide here are focussed on quickly achieving normalisation,' the Professor suggested.

'Normalisation?' John queried.

'Yes. the principles of normalisation are achieved through living a normal life, in a normal environment without heavy dependency on drugs.'

'Hence the sheltered housing?' John suggested.

'Exactly. I believe that it's an important step for their recovery following their treatment regime,' the Professor concurred.

'Do you mean as a result of whatever treatment method that had involved? John queried.'

'Let's assume that we are talking about the present, chemical treatment methodology,' the Professor suggested forcefully.

'OK,' John capitulated, fearful of pushing his viewpoint too far at this early stage.

'Then we're looking for a gradual easing into a normal way of life with a minimum of bureaucratic restraint,' the Professor explained. 'Which of course can't be risk free.

'No, there are always hidden dangers around the corners of everyday life,' John volunteered. 'Do you mean allowing our clients to be able to take the risks?'

'Yes. And clearly with that freedom comes social responsibility. Sometimes that is the hardest thing for our clients to adapt to and deal with. Some cope with it better than others. In fact we have one female who can be quite violent.'

'Really?' John's imagination conjured up a Boadicea character.

'Yes, you'll meet Marilyn soon, I've no doubt. She is usually Eddy's constant companion.'

'I didn't see her on the ferry.'

'No, I gather she doesn't like boats, but that's probably the only time they are apart.'

'Oh.'

'Anyway we give then free rein and attempt to manage any problems that our clients create, especially within the local community, with timely intervention,' the Professor expanded.

'I've a similar mindset,' John observed. 'To allow people to play with fire, provides them with a valuable lesson, if they subsequently get 'burnt'. Although I recognise that some 'fires' can be more serious than others.'

'Exactly. I'm glad we are thinking along similar lines,' the Professor beamed. 'I think I've made a wise choice employing you.'

'I look forward to working with you as well.'

'Me too,' the Professor replied extending his hand.

John stood and shook the other's hand firmly.

'So where do you think Mental Health science will lead us in the future?' John quizzed.

'I believe there is one single cause for all mental health issues. And someday soon, I hope to prove it,' the Professor revealed passionately.

Chapter Nine

After meeting with the Professor and discussing his new role, John was feeling buoyed up and pleased that he had made the right choice of coming to Australia.

With a spring in his step, he quickly made his way back down to reception. Laura looked up as he arrived.

'Everything Ok?' she asked hesitantly, aware that several other previous job applicants had failed to warm to the Professor and decided that the job wasn't for them after all.

'Yes, fine thanks. I think I'll enjoy working here,' he said smiling.

'Oh so pleased to hear that,' Laura beamed. The Professor's not a bad old stick but he can be a bit pedantic. Beware he's a workaholic, he expects big commitment from his people.'

'Thanks for the warning. If there's something interesting going on, I can be a bit work focussed myself,' John added.

'Right John, let me take you to your flat so that you can unpack and settle in,' Laura suggested. 'Back to the lift,' she directed.

John picked up his suitcases and followed.

'I'll hold the door open for you to get in,' she said, standing aside with her arm resting against the opened doors to prevent them closing prematurely.

'Thank you,' he said, stepping in.

'All the flats are on floor three,' she explained, pushing the appropriate floor button.

'Do you have a flat here?' John enquired casually.

'No. I live offsite on the other side of town,' she informed him. 'The flats here are only for Doctors so that if necessary they can be quickly in action.'

'The Professor didn't mention that was part of the deal,' John revealed. 'I'm not sure about that.'

'No, and that's why everyone tends to have another place away from here,' she chuckled. 'So they aren't at the Institute's beck and call.'

'Oh that works well then,' he observed. 'But if it's in their contract?'

'Yes you'd think that was the case but it's not. Perhaps I shouldn't be telling you that,' Laura admitted. 'Although the Professor is brilliant in his field, unfortunately his admin is pretty shoddy. Apparently he didn't think it was needed in the employment contract. He assumed that the Doctors would all want to live here, rent free and put up with the occasional inconvenience of being permanently on call.'

'So what happens if they aren't on the premises?' John queried.

'They're called in, but charge a fee,' Laura revealed.

'Cheeky.'

'Yes, I agree. Well one of my jobs is to sort out the admin side of the institute and close loopholes like that,' she explained.

'How long have you been here?'

'Three years, two working for the Professor and I'm enjoying all the challenges that the Institute is giving me. Here we are,' she said, as the lift jolted to a halt. 'It's round this way,' she said leading him along a short, carpeted corridor.

'Oh this looks nice,' he said, admiring the many modern pictures that adorned the boldly decorated wallpapered walls.

'Yes I have to say that they have really gone to town on making it look nice and modern. That large swirly design is pretty eye catching though isn't it? Wait until you see inside the flat,' she said, opening room nine and entering.

'No key?' he queried.

'The key was already in the lock, as it is for all the unused flats,' she informed him.

John followed her in and thankfully put his suitcases down. 'No more lugging those, I hope,' he thought.

'Your key,' she said, offering it to him.'

'Thanks.'

'This is your lounge, she explained showing him around.' Nice big settee, couple of armchairs, coffee table, television.'

He looked around the large comfortably decorated room. There was a big, framed picture of the Sydney harbour bridge on one wall and the conch shell like Sydney Opera house on the other.

'This door leads to the kitchen,' she said, guiding him in to a fully equipped kitchen.

'It's got a cooker, fridge, washing machine, tumble dryer and large work surfaces either side of the sink,' she reported.

'Wow! No excuse for me not to do any cooking then,' he said, looking around.

'Do you cook?' she wondered.

'Yes, I'm quite a good cook, even though I say so myself,' he volunteered.

'Not short on modesty either are you?' she joked.

'I learned to cook at Uni. It was either that or live out of tins or starve. I tell you what, just to prove it, I would love to cook you a meal one day,' he offered.

'Oh yes. That would be nice,' she smiled. 'I hate cooking, I can probably manage to create a salad, but that's all. Anything that gets me out of cooking is just fine by me. I'll look forward to that then and I'll bring the wine.'

'It's a date,' he said, hoping that it might even lead to one.

'Through this door is the bedroom,' Laura said, leading him in to a generously sized room.

'A nice comfortable double bed,' she said prodding it. 'And through that door is the bathroom, complete with shower and bath.'

John opened the door and scanned the bathroom.

'This is very good. Nicely decorated. I'm impressed.'

'Ok, I'll leave you to unpack now. What time did you want to do a tour of the sights?' she asked.

'Are you sure that you want to do it? John asked concerned. 'I felt embarrassed for you. The Professor rather put you on the spot.'

'No I'm more than happy to do that. I usually end up taking Institute visitors around Manly anyway.'

'Well, if you're sure?'

'Yes, perfectly happy. I have to say that the best part of the evening is that we have to visit a restaurant at the end of the tour,' she smiled. 'So again no cooking for me.'

'Well in that case, who am I to say no. I just need a couple of hours shut eye now. So, shall we say seven pm?' he proposed.

'Seven it is. That will allow me to dash home and freshen up too,' she said going to the door. 'I'll meet you outside by the main entrance downstairs. By the way, I forgot to tell you that the Institute doors are locked at five o'clock, but your flat key also opens the side entrance door which is around the corner near the main entrance.'

'Ok thanks,' he said wearily. Now that the euphoria of meeting the Professor was over, he was feeling the effects of his long, tiring, and exciting day.

'See you later,' she said leaving.

John smiled as he picked up his suitcases and went to the bedroom. 'What a great start to the job. A nice welcome and a date as well.'

He set his alarm clock and without undressing, lay down on the bed. Almost before his head hit the pillow, he was fast asleep.

Chapter Ten

The white coated pathologist put down the vibrating bone saw and carefully removed the skull section that he had skilfully trepanned.

With meticulous precision, based on years of experience, he reached into the cranial vault and deftly removed the brain.

Giving the folds and creases of the brain a quick cursory look, he put the pinkish-grey walnut looking organ into a large stainless steel kidney dish.

'That's the third person, this month, associated with the Imagine Mental Health Institute, on whom I've conducted an autopsy,' the pathologist observed, removing his mask. 'All of them have had significant brain damage, as you can see here,' he said to the lawman, pointing to the hole in the brain's frontal lobe.

The police veteran was unphased by the sight and smell of the removed organ, having attended numerous autopsies and horrendous traffic accidents during his twenty year career in the New South Wales police.

'Perhaps their mental illness was caused by the same brain disease that made the hole?' Police Sergeant, Jon Baldy, suggested. 'And I guess that's the reason why they were all at the Manly Imagine Institute in the first place,' he added.

'Maybe. But I think there's more to it than that.'

'Really?'

'Yes. I'd like to investigate a bit further and determine if there's any pharmaceutical link to the cause of these holes.'

'So when do you aim to do that?' the policeman asked.

'No it needs further expert investigation, I'll send samples off for further forensic analysis by my neuropathologist colleague. We should know if my theory is right or not, when the results come back.'

'How long is that likely to take?'

'Six to twelve weeks, if we're lucky,' the pathologist informed him.

'As long as that?'

'Yes I'm afraid so. But in the meantime, I'll sew this one back up. Do you know if there are any relatives?'

'No, I doubt it. Sadly, a lot of the Institute's residents lose their family ties because their ill health often leads to bouts of erratic behaviour.'

'Yes, I can understand that. The stresses placed on their relatives must be enormous.'

'I imagine that it must be like sitting next to a ticking timebomb, never knowing when the next episode will occur.'

'Do we have a name for this one?' the Pathologist asked.'

'Yes, the Institute tell me his name is Digger Lucas,' the Policeman advised.

'Well at least I can give him a bit of dignity by giving his compartment, in the body storage unit, a name.'

'Sad though isn't it? That's probably how he'll be remembered just another statistic from the Institute,' the policeman reflected.

'You know, I'm very suspicious about the other deaths associated with that place,' the pathologist revealed.

'Why do you say that?'

'The Professor at the Institute convinced me that as they were under his professional care, we needn't conduct a fall autopsy,' the pathologist recalled.

'Do you think there might be something underhand going on then?' the Policeman wondered.

'Possibly. But as we both know, it's dangerous to speculate, unless you have hard factual evidence.'

'Too true. So I guess we'll have to await the results from your colleague then?'

'Yes. Do you know any other suspicious circumstances that we should consider? Any commonality?' the pathologist probed.

'Only the sheltered housing complex where they all lived,' the Policeman observed.

'Mmm, perhaps they've all been using a bad batch of the same illegal drugs?'

'Maybe.'

'However, as you are already aware, irrespective of the brain damage, the cause of death for Mr Lucas here, was a knife through the heart. You have a murder enquiry on your hands Sergeant,' the pathologist concluded.

'Yes, I know.'

'Do you have a suspect in mind?'

'Yes, it'll be one of his own from the psychiatric hospital, I predict,' the policeman said, confidently.

'Sounds like you're pretty sure then.'

'Yes. I've got my suspicions about a particular aggressive female patient that might be behind it. I've sent the knife off to the lab for a fingerprint check. So I'll chase it up when we've cross checked our records,' the Policeman explained.

'So, are you going to be arresting her soon?'

'No. I'm quite happy to wait. She isn't likely to be going anywhere, anyway.'

'Well, best of luck with that strategy. Hopefully, we won't have any more bodies from that place.'

'No hopefully not. Anyway at the request of the local council officials we keep a close eye on the sheltered housing and its occupants. What you going to do with matey here?' the Policeman asked.

'Well now we've got a name, he deserves some dignity in death,' the pathologist said, writing Digger's name on the label attached to the corpse's toe and sliding the stainless steel tray into the body storage unit.

Chapter Eleven

Meanwhile in the offices of a local television production company, plans were being discussed for forthcoming programmes.

'Right Sophie, your dodgy Landlords documentary is being broadcast soon. It's in final edit now,' the hippy looking television producer, Sebastian Way, advised her.

'Great. I worked my ass off to flush out those sick perverts,' she reiterated.

'Have you had any fallout from your investigations yet?'

'Oh the usual hate mail and threats to carve me up,' she explained nonchalantly.

'And that's before its broadcast. Obviously, there will be more after, I assume,' the producer observed.

'It's nothing to worry about,' Sophie observed optimistically. 'I get my PA to read them and then bin them. I can't be arsed to give those lowlifes any time of day,' she said dismissively.

'Good for you. Anyway, this new proposal of yours to investigate this Professor chappie, um what's his name?'

'Phillips. Professor Phillips,' the woman clarified.

'Yes, Phillips, that's right. What's the angle?'

'Mental Health drugs scandal, I believe.'

'What proof have you got that he's up to no good?'

'One of my Police sources has tipped me off that something strange might be going on at the sheltered housing complex associated with the Imagine Institute.'

'Imagine Institute! How does this tie up with this Professor chappie?'

'He runs it.'

'Right. And why the suspicions?'

'There has been several unexplained deaths of residents of the complex. All the victims might have suffered the same type of brain damage from the drugs they are taking.'

'Might have?'

'Yes. Obviously, it needs to be verified. But my informant tells me that the pathologist who carried out the autopsies is very suspicious about the causes of death.'

'So what's this got to do with the Professor?'

'I believe he's pumping them full of unlicensed drugs.'

'So you reckon this Professor chappie is playing Frankenstein do you?'

'Yes, I think that he might be using his position as head psychiatrist at the hospital to use the 'residents' as guinea pigs for his research.'

'Got any evidence?'

'No not yet,' she revealed. 'I...err...tried to get some by speaking to one of the patients, but things got a bit...a bit hairy,' she recalled uncomfortably. 'So I'll have to have a rethink.'

'So with no evidence, we could in fact be barking up the wrong tree?'

'Yes, maybe. But it's rumoured that the people who have died were all involved in some sort of trial.'

'Drug trial?'

'Yes.'

'Mmm, is this good TV? I mean does anyone care about these type of people anyway?'

'Probably not. Although surely there's got to be some relatives out there who care about them, don't you reckon?'

'I'm not sure. They're all on the edge of society. Is it really newsworthy?'

'Yes of course. Eminent Professor killing patients! It's a scandal waiting to be exposed,' she replied dramatically. 'I think it is definitely newsworthy and community minded too.'

'Really?' the producer said, sceptically.

'I can see the headlines in the papers the following day. *'Top TV investigator exposes Mental Health patient scandal'*. Oh yes,' she thought.

'OK, but let's hope you can get some meaty stuff before we definitely commit to it,' he insisted.

'I've already started getting to know some of the residents,' she explained.

'Good. That's what I like to hear.'

'We'll be crusading for the vulnerable. And for a few awards, I'd hope,' she thought.

'The networks will like that,' he enthused, warming to her proposal.

'That's what I thought. And our professional standing for documentary making will be enhanced too,' she crowed.

'Although we'll have to be very delicate with it. Some people are a bit sensitive about mental health issues,' the producer observed.

'Yeah, as I've already found,' she agreed, rubbing her bruised arm.

'So how are you going to go about it?' he quizzed.

'There are some anti-psychiatry protest groups which have been making themselves known around the Institute for some time now. I'll join them and infiltrate. They call themselves 'Reject'; Sophie revealed.

'Never heard of them,' the Producer observed.

'It's a protest group against mental health treatments. They believe that there is no such thing as mental health problems anyway. Hence, that the so-called treatments are more damaging than the 'disease' and therefore inhumane.'

'So people who have problems are faking it, is that what they're saying?'

'No they say that it's all down to individual's behavioural traits,' Sophie explained.

'Well you live and learn,' Sebastian admitted. 'So what's your intention of getting into bed with them?'

'They might already have something about the Professor that I can use.'

'Careful with that second hand information though. We don't want to end up with a legal challenge on our hands. Or antagonise people before we've got a story.'

'Yes, well that's another aspect of the story.'

'What's that?'

'The tensions between the local inhabitants and the residents of the sheltered housing complex.'

'So where does this anti-psychiatry mob fit in then?'

'They are protesting against the Professor and the hospital in support of the patients. Whereas the locals are protesting about the 'do-gooders' and....'

'Do-gooders?'

'The anti-psychiatry mob.'

'Yeah I'm with you.'

'…From coming into their neighbourhood with their high moral principles and undermining their case to get the sheltered housing closed down. In reality if they only stopped to think about it, they are both after the same aims.'

'So there's some aggravation there already?'

'Yes. there's a fair bit of tension building,' Sophie confirmed.

'Excellent. Make sure that your crew captures any bit of violence then. That's good for the ratings.'

'Yes, I thought you'd like to hear that,' Sophie smiled, feeling that she'd sold it well and secured the documentary.

'So what do you need to get it off the ground?' the Producer asked.

'I'll disguise myself, so I'll need my usual make-up artist, wigs and prosthetics.'

'Right. But what are we talking about by way of a budget?'

'I'll get back to you on the finances. I'm still doing background work,' Sophie explained.

'But before you go rushing off and plunging headlong in to it, we'll have to see how your landlord's documentary goes down.'

'Why?'

'To gauge if the audiences are ready for this type of exposé.'

'Oh, OK.' Sophie said, disappointed at his caveat.

'But assume that it will go well,' he added positively. 'And carry on anyway. Keep me updated of any progress. Stay safe.'

'Will do.'

Sophie left the office with a spring in her step, happy that her ambitions for continued celebrity was well on course.

Chapter Twelve

Eddy and Marilyn were sitting next to each other on the local park bench. Their favourite spot was only a few minutes away from their bungalows in the sheltered housing complex where they both lived.

As outpatients of the Imagine Institute they were dressed the same as each other in grey track suit tops and jogging bottoms and could easily have been mistaken for brother and sister. They were both slightly overweight and coincidentally the same age, 35.

Since arriving at the Institute from different mental health hospitals, the pair had become constant companions, although their relationship was strictly platonic.

Temperament wise they differed greatly, Eddy was a very sensitive, emotional butterfly and hated violence, whereas Marilyn was the opposite, tough, short tempered and often the instigator of trouble. She had become Eddy's unofficial bodyguard. She saw her role in life as protecting him from the abuse from the local yobs and ensuring that no harm came to him.

'Did you go on your usual trip on the ferry Eddy?' Marilyn asked.

'Yes, I did,' Eddy said, reflectively.

'So did anything interesting happen?'

'A man told me that I wasn't too old to be a doctor,' Eddy relayed excitedly. 'Not like what the Professor had told me.'

'Oh, that's good. But why do you want to be a doctor anyway?'

'I don't know,' Eddy confessed, 'I just do.'

'Do you remember when you were small,' Marilyn asked.

'No. I don't remember much. I sometimes try to remember and...'Eddy replied, furrowing his brow.

'And what ?'

'My head goes...you know...funny,' Eddy revealed.

'Have you got any sweets?' Marilyn said, bored with hearing about Eddy's usual problems with his 'funny' head.

'No, sorry.'

'When I was small I used to love sweets. I kept them in a secret place,' Marilyn informed him randomly.

'A secret place! Why?'

'Cos my brother and sister used to pinch them otherwise.'

'Where did you keep them? Eddy probed.

'I... I can't tell you. It's a secret,' Marilyn said, crossing her arms defiantly across her chest.

'Go on tell me,' he begged. 'Where was your secret place?' I promise not to take your sweets.'

'I suppose it's all right to tell you now anyway, coz it's not there anymore,' the woman explained, irrationally looking around to make sure that there was no one else in earshot. 'My hiding place was in the airing cupboard,' Marilyn revealed.

'The airing cupboard! That's where your secret hiding place was?' he repeated in surprise.

'Yes, but you mustn't tell. Promise.'

'Promise? Okay I promise.'

'Yeah. I used to hide in there too,' she continued.

'Why?'

'To get away from my brother and sister They were horrible to me and called me names and upset me...but I could stay in there a long time because I had my sweets. I could hear them looking for me. But they never guessed I was in there. They just walked by without finding me.' Marilyn revealed triumphantly.

'Clever.'

'But they never said sorry for calling me names and upsetting me either.'

'That wasn't nice.'

'It was their own fault that it happened. I'm not a Dumbo, I'm not,' she blurted.

'What do you mean?'

'My ears aren't big are they? Are they?' she shouted, turning to face him.

'I don't know. I've never seen you without your headband and long hair,' Eddy said, wondering why she was making such a fuss.

'But the airing cupboard isn't there anymore, either,' she continued.

'Why, what happened?'

'The house burnt down.'

'Really?'

'I never meant for it to happen. But they shouldn't have kept calling me those names. They shouldn't, they shouldn't,' she said, suddenly starting to cry.

'Oh. That's terrible...about your house,' Eddy said shocked.

'I only wanted to be like the others. To be their friend. I didn't want them to go away forever,' she sobbed. 'I just wanted them to stop calling me names,' she explained.

Eddy felt uncomfortable at her distress and wondered about putting his arm around her shoulder, but he thought better of it as he knew that she didn't like people touching her.

'What!...I mean... where did they go?' he mumbled.

'I love my mum and dad. I really do,' Marilyn said softly, choking back the tears. 'But they don't love me anymore.'

'Why?' Eddy asked dumbly.

'Because of my brother and sister going away forever,' she said wiping her nose.

'Does your Mum and Dad come to see you?' Eddy asked innocently.

'Have you got any sweets?' Marilyn asked, evading the question.

Chapter Thirteen

At seven o'clock, John was waiting by the main entrance as arranged. He had struggled to wake, but now, suitably showered and wearing casual evening clothes he was looking forward to his guided tour of Manly.

Suddenly next to him a car pulled up. It was a sleek, white, two door Triumph Herald convertible, with the roof down.

'G'day John, ready for a tour of our fair city?' Laura asked.

'Hello Laura. Wow, nice motor,' he said, admiring the car's sleek lines.

'Hop in and we'll go for a spin,' she instructed.

'This is a nice surprise,' he purred as he climbed into the black leather seat.

'Glad you like it. I've had it for about a year now. I've been very pleased with my baby,' she said, stroking the dashboard lovingly.

'So where are you taking me on the tour?'

'It's going to be a bit of a mystery tour around Manly,' she said putting the car into gear and pulling away. 'I'll take you to some places that you might want to revisit later and some places that you might like to avoid because of the tourists.'

'I'm in your capable hands,' he smiled, sitting back.

'Right, where to start? We have such a wealth of things here; there's fabulous beaches if you want to swim, sunbathe or play volley ball; we've got wild life reserves; Aboriginal artifacts. There's lots of water sports, surfing, boating; If you're into it there's fishing in the rivers, sea, reservoirs, or lakes. No matter where you go, you are always near water and marinas.'

'Sounds great,' he enthused. 'I always wanted to live by the seaside.'

'When you got off the ferry did you see the Corso?'

'Not that I'm aware of. What is it?'

'Basically a shopping precinct or Mall. The Corso was built in 1855 as a boardwalk. The street allows tourists to cross the sand spit between the harbour pier and ocean beach. It follows the track worn by the local Aboriginal people between Manly Cove and Ocean Beach.'

'Fascinating.'

'Of course you're going to have to learn to slow down,' she advised.

'Slow down ?' he queried.

'Too true. No more rush and dash. Part of the way of life here is to chill. Go out with friends have a few tinnies and enjoy a barbie.'

'That sounds quite weird. Barbie is a doll in the UK,' he joked.

'Yes, here too,' she gave him a sideways glance, thinking British humour was weird. 'Of course there are traditional fish and chip places too; she added.'

'Who'd have thought it?' he mused.

'Yes, lots of top quality restaurants if you want to eat out; And if you want to go for a run, there's loads of parks. If you're in to walking there is a Manly to Spit coastal walk.'

'Spit?'

'Yes, it's a ten kilometre walk. Attractions include the tidal pool in Fairlight, the Clontarf Beach, Reef Beach and Crater Cove. You can even do whale watching from there during the migration season.

'Sounds fascinating,' he observed.

'Then there's Grotto Point Lighthouse and finally the Spit Bridge.'

'Grotto point! Spit bridge! You do have some funny place names,' he chuckled. 'Whatever, I'm hooked. I shall have to put that walk on my to-do list.'

'You'll see Spit as we go over the Spit bridge later to get to the restaurant,' she explained.

'Such a lot to choose from, I wonder if I'll ever have time to do any work,' he smiled.

'Right answer,' she echoed. 'Pleasure before work, I like your thinking.'

'Perhaps a little bit of work to earn some money to get the work life balance correct,' he admitted.

'Tell me something about yourself,' Laura asked, as they circumnavigated the area.

'Well, where shall I start? I did five years in Medical School for my degree, I did a couple of years foundation, three years core training then another three years to specialise and I majored in hypnotherapy. I always fancied a life down under and now here I am, living the dream,' he enthused.

'It sounds terribly boring all that academic stuff and training,' she observed.

'Could be, but I decided too much studying could make John a dull boy. So I used to drive fast cars as a hobby. In fact I had a racing driver's license and raced BMW's.'

'Oh dear,' she said, suddenly self-conscious. 'So you must think I'm a bit of a slow driver then?'

'No. I think you're doing brilliantly. I wouldn't criticise anyone's road driving. I learnt the hard, and expensive way, about separating road and race track after bending a few road cars.'

'Oops!'

'I always had to wind down after a race otherwise the adrenalin was still pumping when I drove home. Unfortunately, before I learnt the lesson, I trashed a few cars, with costly consequences.'

'Sounds like an expensive lesson. Although, in your profession, I would have expected you to understand the psychology of doing that anyway,' she teased.

'But I'm still human. To err is to...' John joked.

Laura chuckled. 'Yeah Ok..'

'But what about you?' he probed. 'Have you always lived here?'

'No. I'm originally from New Zealand, a place called Christchurch.'

'Yeah, I've heard of it. I thought New Zealand was a lovely place and still enjoying an innocent period avoiding all the trauma's that the rest of the modern world is experiencing.'

'Yes it is. The snow-capped mountains, the glaciers, the lakes, the geysers, the Māori culture. All magnificent,' she confirmed.

'So why leave? It sounds idyllic,' he probed.

'I wanted a bit more out of life,' she stated. 'So I managed to wrangle enough points to get a job here.'

'And are you enjoying your new life?' he asked.

'Too true. It's living up to my expectations. I've made lots of friends here.'

'A beautiful young lady like yourself probably has no shortage of boyfriends either,' he suggested.

'And so to the tour,' she said, quickly cutting him off. 'You've obviously seen the Ferry terminal but here is the main area where some hospital people have their offsite houses or apartments.

'Ooops!' he thought. 'Too early in our relationship to be making delicate observations like that.'

'Once you're settled, you might want to have words with a few house vendors, otherwise you will be forever the doctor on call.'

'Thanks, I'll probably take your advice.'

'The Esplanade is an area which attracts 'high flying' professionals such as yourself.'

'Oh, I wouldn't put myself in that category,' he said modestly.

'Are you into art?' she wondered.

'Not particularly. I can take it or leave it,' he revealed.

'Well we have a lovely art gallery and museum in the cove here in the Esplanade.'

'I'll know where to come for a bit of culture then,' he said, as they drove by the large building.

'And if you want to see a bit of nature, then I'd recommend Cabbage Tree Bay Aquatic Reserve.'

'The what?' he queried, smiling. 'Cabbage Tree!'

'Yes, they reckon there's more than 160 different species of fish in the reserve.'

'Incredible,' he observed, still smiling at the name.

'Anyway, now you have seen some of the sights and we've been driving around for a while, have you got your bearings?'

Yes, I think that I could find my way around now thanks. You're certainly not short of coastline though are you? But all this lovely fresh sea air has made me hungry, let's eat,' John suggested.

'Ok. I'm glad that you said that. I am going to take you to a very special restaurant right on the seafront it's called the Surfers Pavilion. It overlooks Middle Harbour with spectacular views over Balmoral Beach.'

'Balmoral! Scottish royalty eh?' he quipped.

'Well, strange that you should say that, but I gather they do get movie royalty in there from time to time. So you might be right.'

'I've booked a table for two by the large picture windows. It's right on the beach with magnificent views over the sea.'

'Great.'

'As you'd expect it has a large fish element to the menu.'

'That's good, I love fish,' he confirmed. 'Is this where you normally bring your visitors?'

'Yes. The Professor isn't one for socialising, so he gets me to bring his business visitors here. As you can imagine, he doesn't need to ask me twice.'

'Us Doctors can be quite boring and 'up' ourselves, so it must be difficult striking up a conversation with all these deep thinkers?' John suggested.

'No, not at all. The majority of visitors are mainly from the pharmaceutical company. So they're more down to earth and 'normal' anyway.'

'Well thanks,' he feigned offence. 'Not all doctors are anally retentive. Some of us are actually down to earth too.'

'Present company excepted,' she giggled.

'You must be one of the restaurant's best known customers then, if you go there that often?'

'Yes, I think you're right. The staff there greet me as one of their regulars. If we're lucky we might even see some celebrities.'

"Rubbing shoulders with screen stars over dinner, can't be bad. But tonight, we are the celebrities,' he joked.

Chapter Fourteen

Laura steered the car in to a parking space off the Esplanade, right outside the restaurant.

'That's fortunate we found a space here,' she said switching off the engine. 'That big white building behind the palm trees is where we are going.'

'Do you need to pull the top over?' he asked, climbing out and standing by the side of the folded hood.

'No thanks. The weather is going to be fine and the level of car theft here is pretty low,' Laura replied.

'My, that is an old building,' John observed, as they walked towards the restaurant. 'It reminds me of an old Spanish mission.'

'Yes you're probably right. It was actually built in the late 1920's to improve the beach facilities for swimmers, in those days called Surfers. Hence it was a pavilion for Surfers.'

'Fascinating,' he said. 'You're a mine of information aren't you?' Thanks for that background,' he smiled.

They walked side by side into the restaurant and was greeted at the door as they entered.

True to her earlier explanation of her patronage there, the Head waiter greeted her by name.

'Good evening Laura.

'Good evening Robin.'

'We have your usual table by the window for you and your guest, please come this way.'

The head waiter led the way over the polished wooden floor. He deftly helped Laura with her chair and skilfully undid the rolled napkin laying it gently on her lap.

Meanwhile John had taken his seat and placed his napkin on his own lap. He looked around at the lovely restaurant with its floor to ceiling French windows overlooking the adjoining beach.

'The striped blue and white upholstery of the settees were obviously designed with deckchairs in mind,' John thought. 'An interesting way of providing static seating to some of the tables. And these stylish wooden chairs obviously make up the other flexible seating arrangements,' he concluded.

Regimentally lined up on the crisp white starched tablecloths were rows of serviette wrapped cutlery. A small unassuming table lamp adorned the middle of each table.

Nearby a cascading floral arrangement complimented the restaurant's décor with it's kaleidoscope of colours.

'Your waiter this evening is Bob,' the head waiter said, introducing them to a white shirted individual who had just arrived at the table.

'I sincerely hope that you enjoy your dining experience with us this evening,' the head waiter said, leaving them.

'Thank you Robin, I always do,' Laura smiled.

'Good evening. Can I get you some drinks?' the waiter asked.

'I'm driving, so I'll have an iced tonic water please Bob, but what would you like John?'

'Oh I normally drink beer, but as it's a special occasion, I think it's got to be something local. A wine perhaps? What do you recommend?'

'The Chardonnay from the Hunter Valley here in New South Wales has become very popular. Might I recommend the Tyrell's Vat 47. It has a flavour of oaky notes, with a buttery taste,' the waiter suggested.

'Yes that sounds good. I'll have a half bottle. The Professor is introducing me to my future patients, tomorrow,' John explained. 'Sorry clients,' he corrected himself. 'So I need to keep a clear head.'

'I'll take your food order when I come back, if you are ready to order, unless you want more time?'

'No that will be fine Bob, thanks.'

The waiter left to get the drinks.

'What would you like to eat John?' Laura asked, looking at her menu.

'Well as you're a regular, I shall be guided by you. I am not a fussy eater, so whatever you are having I'll have one of the same.'

'Are you sure?'

'Yes. Just order when he comes back,' John suggested. 'Tell me, what exactly is your job at the Institute? If you don't mind me talking about work over dinner.'

'No, not at all. After all the business is paying for this evening. I suppose you could call me a 'girl Friday',' she suggested.

'So you do anything and everything then?'

'Yes, you're probably right. I do everything from receptionist, opening the post, making the tea, secretarial work and the Professors PA.' I quite enjoy the variety, I must confess,' she added.

'And the business's public relations hostess as well, by the sound of it,' he added.

'Yes, I'd not thought of it like that,' she agreed. 'But yes, you're right.'

'Well hopefully you might find some time to help me to acclimatise with the job too.'

'Be more than happy to,' Laura replied, smiling.

Bob returned with the drinks, putting an ice bucket containing the Chardonnay on a small adjoining table and eased out the cork.

'Would you like me to pour Sir?'

'Yes please.'

'Would you like to taste it first?'

'No, I'm quite sure it will be fine, thanks. Just pour.' John directed.

'Have you decided on your meal choice?' the waiter asked as he filled John's wine glass.

'Yes Bob, I'll have the usual,' Laura said. 'A dozen Sydney Rock Oysters, to share, cured duck breast and Swordfish for the main. My guest will have the same. Is that Ok for you John?'

'Yes, it sounds delicious,' he confirmed.

'We'll order dessert later, Bob,' Laura added.

'Ok, thank you,' the waiter confirmed the order and left.

'How come you decided to work at the Institute?' she quizzed.

'Before I applied for the job, I did a fair bit of research into the Professor's work.'

'Very wise. You were obviously impressed?'

'Yes, I was. It looks like he's quite a pioneer in pushing the boundaries of psychiatry. His theories are mentioned in many international medical journals.'

'His worldwide notoriety attracts a lot of media attention too,' Laura explained. 'Oh and I forgot to mention, when we were listing my jobs, that I am also his press secretary.'

'My, you are a busy lady.'

'I hope I'm not breaking any confidences, but he also gets calls from other Professionals, TV, and Radio who are all keen to hear about his pioneering work,' Laura revealed.

'Quite a celebrity then?'

'Yes, although he hates being in the limelight, he considers anything that takes him away from his research. What he calls his real job; is a waste of time.'

'I can understand that. If you are totally focussed on something, any intrusion can be annoying.' John acknowledged.

'However, not all the calls are positive,' Laura added.

'What do you mean?' he puzzled.

'Not everyone is comfortable with Care in the Community. The patients in the sheltered housing are often the target for local yobs. Not to mention the anti-psychiatry brigade who mount protests outside the Institute from time to time. But, then again, it all makes life less predictable, I suppose,' she said reflectively.

'Protesters?' John said, surprised.

'Yes. Between the two of them they don't like us or our clients very much,' Laura explained.

'Well I hadn't seen that one coming,' John said, alarmed. 'The Professor didn't mention anything about that.'

'Don't worry, apart from a bit of placard waving and chanting, they are pretty well behaved. The local yobs tend to be a bit more of a problem though.'

'Thanks for telling me. Forewarned is fore armed,' John said uncomfortably.

The meal arrived and John was suitably impressed by the meticulous attention given to the presentation of the dishes.

'Nice choice Laura, I must say.'

After they'd demolished the oysters and finished the main course. John voiced his satisfaction. 'Lovely food,' he observed.

'I'm glad that you enjoyed it,' Laura said. 'So are you ready for dessert yet?'

'Yes please. If the dessert is as good as that. It will be the crowning glory of a lovely meal, with the exception of the lovely company of course,' he flattered.'

Laura blushed at the compliment.

'You say the nicest things but I can assure you that the dessert will be even nicer. I suggest that we have the sapphire grape granite for dessert.'

'Sounds intriguing, what's in it?'

'Sheep yoghurt, mousse, vanilla milk and meringue. It is heavenly,' she gushed.

After the meal they had a leisurely drive back to the hospital where John wished her a good night.

'Thanks so much for the lovely evening. It has been a brilliant introduction to my new life,' he beamed.

'My pleasure,' she smiled.

'As well as cooking you a dinner, perhaps I can treat you to another meal there sometime?' he suggested boldly.

'Yes…yes of course that would be very nice,' she spluttered. 'Anyway, welcome to the Institute. See you tomorrow.'

As he climbed out of the car, John leant over and gave Laura a peck on the cheek. 'Thank you again,' he smiled.

Laura put her hand up to her cheek and jiggled nervously at the sudden intimacy and blushed.

'Ooops! What was I thinking of? That wines' gone to my head. I shouldn't have kissed her,' he thought, as he watched Laura drive off.

Quickly he let himself in through the hospital side door. 'That's going to be awkward tomorrow,' he thought, as he locked the door.

Chapter Fifteen

The following morning, as planned, the Professor took John on a familiarisation tour of the Imagine Mental Health Institute estate.

'I expect that you've seen enough of wards in mental health hospitals, so we'll do that visit later,' the Professor suggested, much to John's relief.

'I assume most of the doors to the wards are locked to prevent patients wandering?' John queried.

'Yes, that's right. But, where we can, we put them into a sheltered housing complex,' the Professor added. 'Let's go and have a look at that next and hopefully I can introduce you to a few tenant clients while we're there. I'm particularly keen for you to formally meet Eddy Jones, he will be one of your main clients.'

"Ok, look forward to it,' John confirmed.

'Well as you know part of Australia's aim is to decentralise mental health and to move away from institutionalisation. It's something that I've been demanding for years and at last I've been able to persuade the authorities.

As a result they have agreed for me to run a trial using sheltered housing to deinstitutionalise clients, whilst I'm also developing a new form of treatment,' the Professor explained.

'Yes, I read about your pioneering work, which is one of the reasons, I came here to work with you,' John enthused.

'If our trial is successful, then I believe they will conduct a full enquiry and the country will follow our lead. So I am very keen to ensure that it is seen to be effective.'

'Yes, I can appreciate your focus on a positive outcome for the trial,' John concurred.

As they passed through reception, John could hear Laura on the telephone, obviously dealing with a difficult call.

'No I'm sorry, but the Professor is not giving interviews,' she said firmly. 'No we don't want to comment on the death of three former patients.'

Intrigued, the Professor went over to her and mouthed 'who is it?'

Laura put her hand over the mouthpiece and whispered, 'Sophie Mcbid.'

'Oh definitely not. No interviews ever with her,' the Professor reiterated, walking back to John.

'Trouble?' John asked.

'That woman on the phone is after an interview, she is a television investigative reporter out to make a name for herself. She is a very objectionable person and will bend the truth at other people's expense.

She and her crew make documentaries and her style is to over-exaggerate problems, many just petty, minor issues. And then when she gets involved she 'magically' fixes the issues, while the cameras are there. They present her as a hero for the down-trodden.'

'A Robin Hood; A people's hero?' John suggested.

'More like a Ned Kelly figure,' the Professor suggested. 'Instead of crusading to fix things, she has a reputation for being a heartless self-centred career driven woman.'

'Don't hold back on the compliments,' John joked.

'It's alleged that she uses forged documents.'

'Forged documents! Why?'

'To persuade people into telling innermost secrets by saying there is a conspiracy against them by their friends and family. Using these false documents as evidence of the plot. Callously making them doubt the integrity of people around them. But of course, these are the bits that you don't see on the screen.'

'I know the type,' John added.

'So if she's nosing around here, we will need to be vigilant,' the Professor warned. 'On no account allow yourself to be interviewed by her.'

'Ok, thanks for the advice.'

'Right, the nearest complex is not far away' the Professor informed him. 'Far enough to dissuade the clients from coming to the institute to report trivial matters, but close enough for us to keep an eye on them. It's a brisk twenty minute walk that's all.'

'I'm quite happy to walk, no problem,' John confirmed.

'Let me explain what we have as we walk. Each sheltered housing complex consists of twelve bungalows positioned around a square of a small grass park. There are four adjoined houses on three sides of an open area.

The bungalows each have one bedroom; a bathroom with shower, sink and toilet; a kitchen diner and a lounge.'

'A bit like a holiday chalet perhaps,' John observed.

'Possibly,' the Professor agreed. 'The front door opens onto a small hallway linking all the rooms together.

The back door opens onto a small garden. The occupants are encouraged to cultivate the garden and keep the lawn tidy.'

''Horticultural stimulus is good for the troubled mind,' John observed.

'Yes. I particularly wanted that put in the design of the complexes, I had a few battles to convince them it was a good use of the land. They wanted to add additional housing instead.'

'That's the trouble with these developers, they are always keen to maximise their investment in land, irrespective of house owners needs for space,' John observed.

'Anyway, as you'd expect, the clients are encouraged to run their own lives, cook and clean for themselves,' the Professor continued. 'They are given a weekly allowance to buy their own food. Limited laundry facilities are provided by the hospital, but clients have to deliver and collect it from the laundry.'

'What about furnishings?'

'The houses are basically equipped with furniture. They have a bed, wardrobe, sofa, table, two chairs, a tv, electric cooker, small refrigerator and a food cupboard.'

'What about supervision?'

'Supervision is minimal, but security is tight.'

'Why the tight security? Do they fight amongst themselves?'

'Well, yes and no. There is an occasional punch up, as you'd expect with people with conflicting views of the world. And unfortunately we did lose a few of our clients. Two died from pre-existing illnesses from poor lifestyle choices before they joined us here. And one was stabbed,' the Professor explained.

'Oh dear. Was he attacked by one of the other clients?'

'We don't know yet. The Police are still investigating the circumstances, but it would appear the weapon used was his own knife.'

'Suicide?'

'Not likely. He was an aggressive character. Perhaps got into a fight and ended up falling on it. Who knows? That's for the Police to fathom out. Unfortunately, the three were all on my trial,' the Professor explained.

'Oh. Presumably, that has messed your stats up?'

'Yes, indeed. Sadly, they were all on my active group. I wouldn't have minded if they had been on the control group using placebos.'

'You suggested a need for tight security too?' John prompted.

'Yes. Some sheltered housing complexes are close to 'social housing' flats and some of the residents don't like our setup or its occupants.'

'Why?'

'They're envious that the state is looking after our clients whereas the social housing dwellers have to scrape together a living and buy their own stuff, mostly on unemployment pay.'

'Yes, I can see why they'd consider it's unfair. But what are the options? Unless you either have a scheme for our clients to make saleable goods by re-investing the profit or you find them employment. What else can you do? It is difficult,' John empathised. 'Perhaps full integration into society is the only answer?'

'Getting rid of the stigma of mental illness is the ideal solution. But sadly, we have a long way to go before we get that utopian situation,' the Professor announced.

'Yes, I agree.'

'Alternatively we find a cure to the causes of mental illness,' the Professor added with a glint in his eye. 'And we eradicate it altogether.'

'That really is utopia,' John said sceptically.

'No. Just a target to aim for,' the Professor suggested, positively.

Now what about Eddy and his issues?'

'Eddy's no trouble...however, like all of our clients, he tends to get a bit excited now and then ...but he's as you'd expect.'

'What does that mean? As you'd expect?'

'Well let's say that I haven't had many complaints about him....just the usual ones.'

'What's usual?'

'People feeling 'intimidated' by him talking at them.'

'What, just talking to them ?'

'No...it's more like AT them, rather than TO them.'

'Does he have any habits that would upset people?'

'No...he doesn't twitch, spit or shout if that's what you mean?'

'So why the complaints then?'

'Usual biased view of people on Eddy's type of medication. He talks with a bit of a slur, a lisp...but as you know, he's actually quite 'together."

'How long has he been here?'

'Actually here...oh, only a few years, before that he was in a series of homes and institutions. Chemically suppressed.'

'Poor chap,' John thought.

Chapter Sixteen

'Right here we are then,' the Professor said as they arrived at the small ordered sheltered housing estate. 'I'm surprised not to see anyone out. Normally the residents congregate on the benches on the green,' the Professor explained. 'We'll go and see if Eddy is in.'

'Ok, looks like a nice quiet environment for the clients,' John observed, looking around at the small collection of bungalows.

'Yes I think having this configuration of four adjoining houses on three sides of the open square, is a nice way of giving them freedom but at the same time some reassurance that they have each other nearby.'

The pair walked over to the bungalow labelled number six and knocked on the pink painted door.

'Interesting colour scheme,' John thought, 'although I suppose pink is a calming colour.'

After a few minutes Eddy came to the door. As he opened it he instantly recognised John and fearfully backed away into the hallway.

'You!' he said, pointing at John. 'On the ferry. You said 'I wasn't bothering you. Have you come to tell me off?' Eddy asked apprehensively, nibbling his finger nails.

'Hello Eddy, No, don't worry, I've not come to complain,' John reassured him.

Eddy slowly stepped back towards his visitors.

'When we bumped into each other on the ferry the other day, we talked about whether he was too old to be a Doctor or not didn't we Eddy?' John explained to the Professor.

'Yes and you said that I wasn't. But the Professor told me that I was,' Eddy pointed out, looking accusingly at the academic.

'Pardon me for my views. But I see that you two have already come to some agreement about Eddy's future abilities,' the Professor remarked. ' Nevertheless Eddy, let me formally introduce you to Doctor John Masters. John is the new psychiatrist at the Institute and he will be taking over your supervision from me for your future treatment.'

'Oh!' Eddy said, open mouthed, surprised at the change.

'Well formalities over. I'll leave you two to have a chat,' the Professor said departing. 'I expect you can find your way back John can't you?'

'Yes, if not I'm sure that Eddy could direct me. Thank you Professor,' John said, as the other strode off.

Out of the corner of his eye John could see one of Eddy's neighbours, a female, paying attention to them.

'Can I come in and have a chat Eddy?' John asked, hoping to look into the house to assess Eddy's independence.

'S'pose,' Eddy said, standing aside.

John walked along the short entrance hall into the lounge followed by Eddy.

You have a nice home Eddy,' the Psychiatrist observed looking around, impressed by the neat order of the place. 'Do you mind if I sit down?' John asked.

'No. Sit down. That's Ok,' Eddy confirmed.

'Thank you.'

John sat on the settee and Eddy joined him, sitting very close to him as he had done on the ferry. 'Clearly Eddy doesn't understand the concept of personal space,' John thought.

'It's nice to see you again.' John said, sitting back into the soft settee.

'You…you too,' Eddy said nervously, suspicious of the Psychiatrist's intentions.

'I'd like to make an appointment with you to start a new series of treatments,' John explained.

'New treatments? What does that mean?' Eddy asked.

'My professional speciality is hypnotherapy,' John explained, and I'd like to ask you to be one of my special clients to help me test it out.'

'Special! A special client?' Eddy said, enthusiastically.

'Yes that's right, a special client,' John repeated.

Oh, but what is hypno…hypnothingy?'

'Hypnotherapy is where I put you in a trance, it's like a sleep, and I try to help your brain sort itself out, John explained

'Are you going to cut me?' Eddy asked anxiously, sliding away from John.

'No. It's nothing like that. It is quite simple. You just lie down and I speak to you very quietly. No tablets, injections, or surgery,' John explained patiently, and you just go to sleep and I talk to you.'

'But if I'm asleep. I won't hear what you're saying,' Eddy reasoned.

'This is a special kind of sleep where your brain is still listening. When I wake you up after the session, you won't remember anything about the conversation that we've had. Do you understand? John asked.'

'Oh! I think so,' Eddy answered with a furrowed brow that showed he didn't really. 'So how will that help me?' Eddy asked confused.

'Because, from your answers I can find out the best way to make you feel better for a long time,' John explained. 'You would really be helping medical science if you said yes,' John suggested.

'Helping science?'

'Yes? And you will be my special client.' John encouraged.

'I'd like to help science,' Eddy confirmed. 'And become a special client too!'

'So is that Ok if I make an appointment with you?' John checked.

'Oh. Ok. If I'm going to be special,' Eddy agreed, nodding.

'I need to do some preparation before we start, so I'll be in touch soon. Is that Ok?'

'Yes. I'm going to be special,' Eddy beamed.

John let himself out, just as the woman who had watched him earlier emerged from the bungalow next door.

As he walked across the square, John could see the woman at Eddy's door.

'Must be friends,' 'he thought. 'Probably wants to know what has been going on.'

Chapter Seventeen

'Who was that?' Marilyn demanded, pushing open the pink front door without knocking and walking straight into Eddy's house.

''He's the new Doctor,' Eddy explained. 'He's going to make me special,' he beamed.

'How is this Doctor going to make you special?' she demanded, jealously.

'Well actually, he's a psy…chia…trist,' Eddy corrected her, whilst annunciating the word slowly.

'Doctor, Psychiatrist, they're all the same to me,' she said dismissively. 'They all mess with your head, just like that Professor. So what did he say? How is he going to make you special?' she demanded.

'He wants to do some hypno…hypno thingamy on me,' Eddy advised her proudly.

'Hypnothingamy!…do you mean hypnotherapy?'

'Yes. That's it. Hypnotherapy,' he confirmed.

'Hypnotherapy that's like hypnotising people and stuff.' she advised him knowledgably.

'Yes, that's right. He's going to send me to sleep and ask me questions to help…help sort my head out,' Eddy explained awkwardly.

'Oh, I wouldn't let him do that to you,' she warned dramatically.

'Why?' Eddy asked concerned.

'I saw a hypnotist at a fair once. He got people from the audience to go on to the stage and he hypnotised them.'

'What happened?' Eddy asked, alarmed.

'He turned them into chickens,' Marilyn revealed dramatically.

'Chickens! What do you mean, chickens? How did he do that? ' Eddy queried, now worried.

'He walked in front of each of them, looked them in the eyes and said something to them. And they all became sort of stiff.'

'Stiff?'

'Yeah and they all started staring in front of them. He then told us in the audience that they were all hypnotised.'

'Hypnotised! And they were stiff and staring?' Eddy repeated.

'Yeah. Then he said to all of them, when I say the magic word *'HENRUN'* you will all become chickens.'

'Chickens! No he didn't!' Eddy dismissed her claim.

'Yes he did,' she argued. 'And then he said *'HENRUN'*, and they all did.'

'What? Become chickens? Never!"

Yes. They started walking around the stage like chickens, making clucking noises and flapping their arms like wings. Marilyn said, demonstrating the chicken strut.

'Oh crikey,' Eddy said, apprehensively chewing his fingers.

'And then he said, I want you to lay an egg.'

'What! People lay an egg? Never!'

'Yes he did,' Marilyn confirmed conspiratorially.

'Did you actually see them lay any eggs?' Eddy asked naively.

'Well the hypnotist showed us a box of half a dozen eggs. He said that he'd picked them up from off the stage,' Marilyn relayed convincingly.

'So are these people still chickens?' Eddy asked nervously.

'No, of course not,' she said dismissively.

'How did he stop them then?'

'He said when I clap my hands, you will become yourself again. And he went 3 – 2 – 1 and clapped his hands. And they all 'woke up' and became themselves again.'

'Oh that's alright then. But I don't want to be a chicken in the first place,' Eddy said firmly.

'But we could have free eggs for breakfast every day,' Marilyn giggled.

'I'm not laying eggs,' Eddy shuddered at the thought.

'But that's not all,' she continued.

'Why, what happened then?'

'So they all went back to their seats and when they'd all sat down, he said *'HENRUN'* and they all immediately stood up and started acting like chickens again. It was ever so funny.'

'Oh in that case, I won't let him do hypnotherapy on me after all,' Eddy said defiantly.

'No, I wouldn't either,' Marilyn agreed cunningly. Pleased that Eddy wasn't now going to have any special treatment that she wasn't also going to be receiving.

Chapter Eighteen

When John got back to the hospital, he popped in to see the Professor to update him. Taking his cue from the previous visit with Laura, he knocked and waited to be invited to enter.

'Come,' came the instruction from within.

John entered the office. The Professor looked up as he entered.

'Hello John, how did you get on with Eddy?'

'Fine thanks. I hope you don't mind but I plan to conduct a hypnotherapy session on him.'

'For what reason?' the academic queried, mildly annoyed that John was still intending to go ahead with hypnotherapy in spite of their earlier discussion.

'To help him to regress and identify any buried anxiety,' John explained.

'I don't think that's a wise course for Eddy,' the Professor counselled.

'May I ask why? John asked, slightly taken a back at the others reticence.

'I'm sorry if this offends you and your beliefs about hypnosis but, I don't hold with that fairground charlatan stuff,' the Professor dismissed.

'Really!' John said, bristling. Astounded at the others directness.

'This man has long term complex mental health issues,' the Professor revealed. ' You can't just magic them away with your 'snake oil' hypnosis.'

'It's not fairground hypnosis. It's real science,' John rebutted the others put-down.

'Real science is all about finding the right medical solution, like in my trial,' the Professor suggested firmly.

'I dispute that,' John argued, spurning the others observation. 'Hypnotherapy is a type of alternative medicine in which hypnosis is used to create a state of focused attention and increased suggestibility,' John recounted passionately. 'During the process positive suggestions and guided imagery are used to help individuals deal with a variety of concerns and issues. Many deep seated.'

'Thank you for the lecture. But I do know what the definition of hypnotherapy is,' the Professor replied testily.

'Yes, sorry, apologies,' John said realising he had been slightly indiscreet in his firm defence. I wasn't trying to teach 'granny to suck eggs',' he grovelled.

'Apology accepted. 'But it doesn't change my view of its effectiveness. I believe that the brain deals best with chemical stimulants, which is why I focus my research in that area,' the Professor said firmly. 'Strictly between you and I, my research is uncovering some interesting findings in 'mind altering' drugs based on hallucinogenic, psychedelic and MDMA compounds.'

'MDMA?'

'Methylenedioxymethamphetamine. Better known as Ecstasy,' the Professor amplified.

'But of course,' John confirmed his understanding. 'Well I look forward to discussing it with you on a more detailed level in the future.'

'Be delighted to. But not about hypnotherapy,' the Professor added quickly.

'I don't understand. I thought you recruited me for my hypnotherapy skills. But now you don't want me to use them? Please explain.' John demanded, incredulous at the other's apparent change of his suitability for the role, unable to hide his disappointment.'

'No. Nothing has changed,' he confirmed. I recruited you for your intellect and vision. Which you have demonstrated by acquiring a hypnotherapy skill, as well as your psychiatry qualifications. This indicates to me that you are a farsighted person. You are the sort of person that I need to ensure my work continues to a successful conclusion,' the Professor explained.

'Then, we'll have to agree to disagree,' the hypnotherapist said, 'sticking to his guns'. 'I have a proven record of success using hypnosis and talking therapy with previous patients.'

'Congratulations. I am pleased to hear it. But I'd prefer that you didn't use it here,' the Professor said firmly. 'Especially on Eddy.'

'Where can I obtain Eddy's records?'

'After what I have just said about Eddy? Why do you want to see them?' the Professor asked, clearly uncomfortable at John's request.

'So that I can have a shot at finding the best way into his psyche.'

'The records are kept in a centralised record office. However I would prefer, at this early stage, that you concentrate on getting up to speed in the processes of the Institute, before you wade headlong into treating Eddy,' the Professor directed. 'Currently he is part of my trial and I don't want any variations in his treatments to distort my data. If you wouldn't mind,' the academic demanded, politely.

'Ok. I get where you're coming from,' John acknowledged. 'No, I won't do anything to ambush your trial.'

'Thank you. I appreciate that. In which case you might be interested in part of my current research.'

'Yes I am always interested in innovation,' John explained.

'I've identified periods of cranial growth and development where adolescents brains become pliable and are forming new connections.'

'How does this help?'

'Well if we can replicate this pliable period in adult's brains, we can introduce a fast acting drug during this critical window, which can help the formation of healthier connections,' the Professor enthused.

'To what end? What are you anticipating will happen?'

'These better connections will mean better cranial pathways. Thus improving patient's mental health,' the Professor gushed.

'Interesting thesis,' John admitted, but still annoyed at the Professors views on the effectiveness of hypnotherapy.

'Yes I think so too,' the academic said enthusiastically.

'However, we appear to have fundamental and conflicting views on some mental health treatments,' John suggested.

'So you think my lifetime's work has been a waste of time then? All my research and treatment developments to help mental health patients worthless?' the Professor challenged, angrily.

'No, I'm not saying that at all. But...'

'How dare you suggest that my drug solutions are bogus,' the Professor interrupted.

'I'm not saying that at all. Like all developments, clearly your research has provided a foundation for others to follow. Subsequent improvements in technology and innovation will enable them to achieve improved results.'

'So you think that all patients would benefit by your circus performance hypnosis do you?' the Professor said, red faced at the others impudence.

'No I'm not. I am saying that some people might benefit, but not all. I recognise it is not a panacea for everything. Different mental health issues need different treatments just like all other health ailments.'

'So you accept that I might be right? And you are gracious enough to allow me to carry on?' the Professor said, sarcastically.

'Yes. But I want Eddy to come off the trial, so that I can wean him off his drugs.'

'And at the end of it; if it doesn't work? Are you prepared to risk the permanent damage that you will cause him?'

'No I don't accept the hypothesis or inevitability that it might not work. I've used my proposed technique, previously with successful outcomes.'

'Eddy has been on medication all his adult life,' the academic argued. 'What you see is a medically managed Eddy. If you take away the thing that is a controlling factor, you are risking his future mental health. Now, at the moment, his life is stable and predictable.'

'I am prepared to take that risk. I've seen glimpses of his behaviour which encourages me to normalise his mental health through hypnotherapy.'

The Professor picked up his pen and returned to his report. A clear signal that their conversation was over.

John took the hint and decided that there was no point discussing the issue any further. He left the Professor's office, deflated, but determined to go ahead with Eddy's hypnotherapy treatment anyway.

He kicked himself for upsetting his new boss so soon into his employment. 'It doesn't bode well for a long term future here,' he thought.

Chapter Nineteen

In addition to questioning passengers on the Manly ferry about whether he was too old to be a Doctor or not, Eddy also paid a regular visit to the local hospital's Accident and Emergency department, where he offered to help. Often just moving wheelchairs and stretcher trolleys into a storage area and generally tidying up rubbish.

His offers were tolerated in a sympathetic way - for a brief period during each visit. But his presence eventually became a nuisance and he was ejected.

'What is it today Eddy? Have you come to do heart surgery? Or a kidney transplant perhaps?' the Nurse asked him, playfully.

'No, I've just come to help you; I heard that you are short of staff. I can see that there are long queues of patients waiting to be seen. Would you like me to do some bandages for you?' Eddy asked the charge nurse, whilst studying the large number of seated casualties.

'No, I think we can cope Eddy. But thanks for your kind offer,' the nurse replied, walking away from him.

'But there are lots of people waiting,' Eddy pointed out.

Undaunted by the charge nurse's rejection of his offer, Eddy approached an elderly lady clutching a bloody cloth wrapped around her finger.

'Excuse me lady, do you want me to put a bandage on your finger?' Eddy asked earnestly.

The woman looked at him in horror and moved away.

The nurse spotted the situation and went back to Eddy.

'Now come on Eddy, if you want to help, just sit there quietly,' she instructed.

'But I want to help you with your queue,' he explained earnestly, looking at her with doleful eyes.

'Yes, I know you do. But not today, eh? As you can see we are very busy.'

The nurse wandered back to reception and said, 'Eddy's back again, get security to do their usual escort job, please.'

'Ok.'

Within a few minutes two uniformed guards arrived in the casualty department and went over to Eddy.

'Come on then Eddy. I think it's time for you to leave now. You've done enough for today.'

'No, I haven't helped at all,' he explained. 'They are so busy, I just wanted to help.'

'Yes I know you do, but I think you need to leave,' they said, gently holding each arm. 'Come on blue.'

Reluctantly, Eddy allowed himself to be escorted off the premises.

'I only wanted to help,' he said under his breath. 'What did Doctor John say that if I allowed myself to be hypnotised I would be helping. Right, that's what I'll do then. If they don't want me here.'

Eddy left the A & E department and went straight to the Institute.

He was greeted by Laura at reception.

'Hello Eddy. What can I do for you?' she asked.

'I would like to speak to Doctor John, please.'

'Is he expecting you?'

'No. Yes. I don't know,' he said confused, trying to fathom out if the Doctor was expecting to hear from him or not.

'Just a minute, I'll see if I can contact him on his pager,' Laura informed him.

'Thank you.'

'Would you like to take a seat while I page him?'

'Yes thank you,' he confirmed and sat on the lounge settee nearby.

Laura dialled the number of John's pager and within a few minutes he telephoned her.

'Reception, how may I help?' she announced.

'You paged?' John replied.

'Yes John. Eddy is down in reception and would like to speak to you.'

'Ok, I'll pop down.'

Within five minutes John walked in to reception.

'Hello Eddy. I gather that you want to see me?'

'Yes. I...I...been thinking. 'I'd like to help you, but I'm scared.'

'Oh, that's good news that you want to help me. Thank you. But why are you scared; may I ask?'

'Well Marilyn said that hypnotherapists turn people into chickens. And I don't want to be a chicken.'

'Chickens!' John puzzled. 'Oh she is probably talking about fairground hypnotists,' John suggested.

'Yes, that's right. Fair ground,' Eddy confirmed.

'Well I don't do that sort of hypnosis. I use hypnotherapy to help people. Just like a Doctor who prescribes various drugs and treatments to cure patients when they are poorly. I use hypnosis instead.' John explained patiently.

'Oh! Well...I...I'd like to help people. And besides they don't want me in A & E,' he explained. 'And you said I'd be special too?'

'Yes you'd be a special person, as I'd said, if you'd help me,' John encouraged.

'A special person...I'd be a special person?' Eddy repeated, running the words through his mind. 'Promise?'

'Yes, like I told you,' John confirmed.

'Oh, Ok. Yes...yes I will. I'll help you then,' Eddy agreed, smiling.

'That's excellent news Eddy. Thank you for volunteering.'

Conscious that Eddy might change his mind again, John suggested an early appointment without delay. 'Shall we say tomorrow at 1100 o'clock?'

'Do you want me to write that time down Eddy?' Laura volunteered, overhearing their conversation.

'Yes please,' Eddy confirmed.

Laura wrote the date and time on a card and gave it to him.

'That's great Eddy. As I said, you will really be helping medical science,' John informed him. 'I'll see you tomorrow then.'

'No chickens?' Eddy checked.

'No. No chickens,' John reassured him.

Eddy strutted out of reception clutching the card, feeling important and very pleased with himself.

'I wonder what brought on his change of mind? Initially he was telling me he didn't want to do it because he didn't want to be made into a chicken,' John revealed.

'A what?' Laura said in surprise.

'It's a long story. I'll tell you over dinner one night,' he said. 'By the way don't mention my appointment with Eddy to the Professor, he's a bit anti hypnotherapy at the moment.'

'Ok. Mum's the word.'

Chapter Twenty

The following day, Eddy checked the card that Laura had given him and the time on his wristwatch, both said eleven o'clock.

He was nervous as he arrived outside John's consulting room for his appointment. He knocked hesitantly but was immediately invited into the small, well equipped, room that smelt of disinfectant.

'Hello Eddy, thanks for coming.'

'Hello,' Eddy said nervously, standing rooted to the spot.

'Come on in,' John encouraged.

Eddy didn't move.

'I know that you have concerns, that's quite understandable. But don't worry. Come on in. I promise I won't hurt you,' John encouraged

'Ok,' Eddy said, apprehensively walking slowly into the room, glancing nervously around.

'Now, if you'd like to sit there on the couch,' the psychiatrist indicated.

Eddy looked suspiciously at the long black leather psychiatrist's examination couch and touched it cautiously.

'It's Ok. It's just an ordinary examination couch. If won't bite you,' John reassured him.

But just as he was going to sit down Eddy spotted something that did frighten him.

'What's that funny hat with the wires sticking out?' Eddy asked anxiously.

'It's an Electroencephalograph cap,' John said casually.

'A what?' Eddy queried.

'We call it an EEG cap for short. It's used as an electrophysiological monitoring device to record electrical activity of the brain.'

'Of my brain?' Eddy asked putting his hand up to his head.

'Yes. Your brain or anyone else that wears it,' John explained.

'How does it work?' he asked suspiciously.

'It goes on your scalp and monitors your brain activity. Don't worry, it's a non-invasive way of seeing what's going on in your head.'

'Really? What's going on inside my head! How does it do that. Are there any pictures?

'No. No pictures. All will become clear shortly,' John said patiently.

'Have you got to cut me though?'

'No. No cutting involved as I said. See these,' John said, picking up the cap and exposing a series of pads inside the cap.

'Yes. What are they?'

'These are things called electrodes.'

'Electrodes?' Eddy repeated curiously.

'The cap places the electrodes around your head and they rest on your scalp.'

Eddy put his hands on his head and felt his scalp.

'The cap makes sure that they are in the right place over parts of your brain,' explained John patiently.

'Over my brain,' Eddy repeated, feeling the shape of his skull, something he'd never thought about before.

'The electrodes are connected via these different coloured wires to this computer,' John said, pointing to a large desktop computer.

'So what does the computer do?'

'It translates the electrical signals from the cap and shows your brain waves on this screen,' John said, patting the huge monitor.

'Oh, I'm not sure that I want to wear that cap,' Eddy said, standing back, nervously twisting his fingers.

'There's nothing to worry about,' John reassured. 'Look, I'll put it on myself and you can see that nothing bad happens.'

And so saying, John put the cap on. He clicked several keys on the computer which then displayed some squiggly green lines on the monitor.

'See nothing is happening to me. It's perfectly safe,' he encouraged. 'All I'm going to do is to ask you lots of questions and I'll be able to see what happens to your brain through all these wires.'

'Oh... Ok,' Eddy said, hesitantly.

John removed the cap from his own head.

'But in order to relax you, I am going to hypnotise you first. Is that alright?'

'You're not going to turn me into a chicken are you?' Eddy checked.

'No. No of course not,' John chuckled.

'Only Marilyn said she saw a hypnotist and he turned people into chickens and they laid eggs.'

'Yes, you've already told me. No Eddy, I assure you that turning you into a chicken is the last thing on my mind.'

'Ok. Are you sure?' Eddy queried, still uneasy about it all.

'Yes, now don't worry. I promise that I won't hurt you. I'd like you to drink this medicine first, it will help to relax you.'

'Why?'

'Because I can see that you are very tense at the moment.'

Eddy looked suspiciously at the proffered glass. It was half filled with a colourless liquid.

'It won't hurt you, I promise,' the psychiatrist assured him.

Eddy finally reached out and took the glass which he smelt before hesitantly tipping it up and drinking its contents.

'That wasn't too bad was it?' John said, taking the empty glass from him.

Eddy shook his head. 'No. It just tasted like water,' he said.

'Right I'm going to put this cap onto your head,' the psychiatrist said, picking up the small skull cap festooned with the coloured leads.

'You're not going to electrocute me are you?' Eddy nervously asked backing away.

'No of course not.'

'Only Marilyn said that Doctors used to zap people's heads with electric and it made them like zombies.'

'No, rest assured. It will be nothing like that. I shall not be applying any electricity through these wires. In fact, quite the opposite. I shall be reading the electrical signals coming from your brain. Is that Ok?'

'I...I suppose so. Are you going to shave my hair off first? Because I like my hair.'

'No, your hair is safe from the clippers,' John reassured him.

Finally Eddy relaxed and sat on the edge of the couch while John fitted the EEG cap gently on to Eddy's head.

Satisfied it was on correctly, he invited Eddy to lie back on the elevated couch.

Chapter Twenty-one

Eddy shuffled along on the couch and lay still.

'I shall ask you a few questions just to make sure that it's working correctly,' John explained, adjusting a few knobs on the monitor.

'Ok.'

'Is your name Eddy?'

'Yes. But you already know that. Why are you asking me?' Eddy queried.

'Just to make sure that everything is working Ok,' John assured him.

'Oh! OK.'

'I'm now going to relax you further,' John explained, sitting alongside Eddy facing him.

'You mean hypnotise me? Remember I don't want to be a chicken, you promised,' Eddy repeated his concern. Suddenly he sat up and stared at John. 'Your eyes!'

'What about my eyes?'

'They remind me of someone,' Eddy puzzled.

'OK, now lie back again. Now don't think about anything else. I promise that you won't be a chicken.'

'You promise?'

'Yes. Now just lie perfectly still and listen to my voice. I want you to relax... relax...relax,' John said quietly in a dreamy sort of voice. 'You will feel your eyelids getting heavy, so very heavy and it's Ok to close them. Just concentrate on my voice. You will still be able to hear me and you will be able to speak. Just relax. That's right. Relax. Let all the tension out of your body. You will feel very light, very light.' John's voice became a quiet whisper, so that Eddy had to concentrate hard to hear.

The monitor showing the EEG readout indicated that Eddy was in a trance. Satisfied with the stabilised line, the psychiatrist asked, 'Is your name Edward Jones?'

'Yes.'

A positive reaction on the screen.

'Ok, I want to take you back to your earliest memory…back to when you were a toddler. Take the journey back Eddy. Back…back through the years,' he encouraged quietly. 'Imagine that you are an observer watching little Eddy, tell me all about him.'

There was a slight pause in Eddy's reaction which concerned John, until at last he spoke in a surprisingly clear voice.

'Eddy, his father and step-mother came to Australia on a big ship. They lived in a big house on the outskirts of Sydney. He was very happy.' They all loved Australia.

John was encouraged by the early signs of Eddy's recall.

Can Eddy recall their names?'

'His Daddy was Justin and his wife was called Beverley. Beverley was Eddy's step mum.'

'Does Eddy keep in touch with his real Mother?'

'No. He doesn't know who she is. His Daddy never spoke about her.'

What did his Daddy do in Australia?

His Dad was a GP. But when he wasn't working his Dad and Eddy went camping and fishing.

'At this point, Eddy became restless. The brain traces becoming erratic.

'Ok Eddy. Don't worry, just relax. Let's go to a happy place. What did Eddy do to make him happy?

'Fishing. He used to go fishing with his Daddy. 'Then Eddy became tense again. 'Oh no. I don't want to say. No it hurts to remember.'

'Why doesn't Eddy want to say? He's safe here. Remember he's in his happy place.' John encouraged.

'No. he can't. He doesn't want to.'

'Eddy's EEG trace was going haywire again.

'Did something happen when he was fishing?' the psychiatrist probed.

'No...no I don't want to remember.' Eddy croaked, thrashing around on the couch.

'Ok. You are obviously resisting, so we'll call it a day for now.' John said disappointed at the brevity of the session and reluctantly brought Eddy out of his trance.

John had been hoping to try and tease out more information from Eddy to understand the background to his situation.

'Ok Eddy. I think we've done enough for today. I'm going to bring you back to the present. Just relax, let your mind be free again. And when you're ready open your eyes. They will feel light again. That's right, slowly open them,' John encouraged.

Eddy stirred and slowly came out of the trance.

'That's good Eddy. When you're ready, sit up and I'll remove the cap. How do you feel?'

'Ok, I think. What happened? Did I help? Did you find out about my illness?'

'It went Ok. Yes you were a great help. But we're not there yet. I think we will need several more sessions to get to the bottom of it,' John said, removing the skull cap.

'Can I go now?'

'Yes of course. You see it didn't hurt did it?'

'No.'

'And as I didn't turn you into a chicken, perhaps we could have another session this time next week?'

'Ok,' Eddy confirmed nonchalantly.

'By the way, you have a bit of an unusual accent it's not quite Australian. The way you sound your R's, sounds like you have an English West Country accent.' John observed.

'Have I?'

'Yes.'

'Oh.'

'Until next week then,' John said, letting Eddy out.

'Well it looks like you have some very deep issues there Eddy,' John thought, as he completed his notes. 'Unfortunately, this may take some time to get to the bottom of it. But the hypnotherapy is bypassing that drugged part of his brain and has triggered his memory and amazingly, as Eddy's observer, he talks with a different and mature vocabulary.

Chapter Twenty-two

John had been trying to work up courage to apologise to Laura for giving her a peck on the cheek after she'd taken him sightseeing around Manly. His indiscretion was so out of character. He was mortified at his lapse. Finally he found an opportunity when Laura was alone.

'Umm, Laura I'm glad I caught you. I...I...err...I am so embarrassed,' John told her, unsure of what reaction he would receive.

'Embarrassed! Why?' she asked, non plussed.

'Well, when you dropped me off the other day, after we'd been sightseeing, the wine and jet lag had obviously affected my usual reserve. I took a liberty and gave you a kiss. I'm sorry if I overstepped the mark,' John said awkwardly.

'Oh, that was nothing. I didn't think anything of it,' she lied, recalling that she felt quite excited by the sudden show of emotion.

'Thank you for being so understanding,' John said relieved.

'Anyway, I was thinking of going for a picnic and swim tonight after work. I've got enough for two if you wanted to join me,' she offered hopefully.

'Well, I...err...I haven't got any plans,' he said, wrong footed by the invitation. 'But I...I don't want to impose. What about your friends?'

'I hadn't arranged anything with anyone in particular,' she lied, thinking that Angela wouldn't mind being dropped for her getting a chance of male company. After all, Angela had been constantly nagging her to find a man anyway. 'That's it then. I've got enough tinnies in the car. Have you got any shorts?' she asked

'Yes, upstairs in my flat,' he heard himself saying.

'Ok, I know a nice quiet little cove that we can go to. Shall we say out front at 5pm?' she suggested. 'I'll drive.'

'Ok, I'll look forward to it,' he beamed.

So rather than making a bad impression on Laura, he was surprised that he had clearly done the opposite.

Later, as he retrieved his swimming shorts from his flat, John had second thoughts about the picnic. 'Should he be fraternising with the staff?. No, probably not. He was already in the Professor's bad books. Although she did take me around Manly. And it's only a picnic after all,' he argued with himself. 'Just another sightseeing opportunity, that's all. There's no harm in it.' He persuaded himself. 'Damn it,' he thought 'I could do with a bit of fun.'

As agreed, the pair met up at five, Laura drove round to the front of the building. As she parked alongside John, he was surprised to see a surfboard on top of the convertible.

'I see you've managed to get your 'board' on the car,' he said sliding into his seat.

'Yes a friend of mine made up a special contraption for me to carry it on my car even though it's a soft top,' she explained.

'Brilliant idea,' he acknowledged. 'Where are we going?' John asked as they drove off from the Institute.

'It's on North Head. The beach is relatively secluded. I love to go there and chill. It's usually tourist free too.'

'This scenery is all new. I don't recognise any of it from our sightseeing the other day,' he said, studying the countryside as they drove through the outskirts of Manly.

'No, we didn't come to this area on our previous sightseeing visit,' she informed him.'

'So what's this place we're going to? Has it got one of those weird names that seems to be prevalent around here?' he teased.

'It's called Quarantine Beach,' she announced, sneaking a sideways glance at him, expecting some comment at the name.

He didn't disappoint. 'Quarantine beach. Is that what I think it is?'

'What do you think it is?'

'Somewhere where they put people with dreadful diseases, like a leper colony?'

'No, not quite. But it is named after the old Quarantine Station which operated from 1828 there until the present day, although I think it is closing soon. It was the first port of call for all quarantined ships and any sick passengers.'

'Do we have to prove that we are disease free then?' he joked.

'No, I think we'll be alright,' she reassured him. 'Anyway as a doctor you could give us both a certificate of good health,' she teased.

After the short journey they arrived at their destination and Laura parked the car. Together they unloaded the bags containing the picnic and bathing stuff out of the small boot.'

'At the risk of being accused of misogyny would you like me to carry the surfboard down to the beach?' John asked cautiously.

'Yes please. I have no objections at all. I'm not a feminist.'

'My! Isn't this great?' John said, taking a deep breath. 'The smell of the sea and the sound of lapping waves caressing the shore makes me feel quite lyrical. Sun and sea. What could be better than that?

'Gorgeous isn't it?'

Together the pair walked the short distance from the carpark on to the beach. John was overwhelmed with the beauty of the place. 'Clear blue sea and white sands. This is seriously impressive,' he said.

'So you like it?' she asked.

'Do I ever.'

'There's lots to do, you can swim, snorkel, kayak, bush walk or simply relax on the quiet beach. Many people come here by boat, and as there are no hidden rocks you can land right on the beach too,' Laura explained.

'It's a big bit of sand.' John said, as they entered the white sandy beach.

'Yes, it's over a third of a mile long. Lovely isn't it?'

'It's obviously a best kept secret there's not many others on it either,' John observed.

'No, and that's why I love it,' Laura said, putting her bags down and digging in to her beach bag and retrieving a large towel.

'I'll put this down so we can lay our stuff on it without it getting covered in sand.' she explained.

Having done so, she quickly removed her shorts and tee shirt, revealing a stylish one piece pink bathing costume on her slim shapely figure.

John tried to be discreet and averted his eyes as Laura slipped out of her clothes. But he found himself ogling as she gently applied suntan lotion to her bronze arms and long legs.

John soon realised that he was not so pre-prepared for the beach as Laura. Feeling slightly embarrassed at his lack of forethought, he sat on the big beach towel and covered himself with a towel loaned from his room.

After a struggle he modestly removed his trousers and underpants, finally slipping his swimming shorts on and removing his shirt.

He was pleased that he kept himself reasonably fit as he exposed his muscular chest.

'Do you want some suntan lotion?' she asked, offering him a bottle.

'Yes please, I suppose I ought to,' he agreed, taking it from her.

'Would you mind putting some on my back too?' she asked. 'I can normally do my shoulders myself but there's always a bit that I miss…and then I'll do yours, if you'd like. The sun is very strong down here in Oz and otherwise you'll get sunburn before you know it,' she counselled. 'Sadly there are a lot of skin cancer cases around here too.'

'OK,' he said taking the bottle and pouring a small amount in the palm of his hand, meanwhile Laura turned round to allow him to access her back, slipping the shoulder straps of her bathing costume off as she did so.

John rubbed his hands together to spread the suntan lotion between them and tentatively touched Laura's shoulders.

It had been many years since he had done the same for his partner and his animal instincts were aroused as he gently massaged Laura's smooth skin.

After a few minutes he reluctantly stopped applying the lotion.

'I think that's all covered,' he forced himself to say having enjoyed the intimacy of touching her. Although still feeling a bit uneasy at the speed of the closeness of their relationship.

'Ok, turn around and I'll do yours then,' she instructed, pouring the lotion in her cupped hand.

Laura was much more business-like in her application to his back, and to his disappointment, had completed the task in no time.

He took the bottle off her and quickly applied suntan lotion to the rest of his body.

'Right, now that's done. 'Come on, I'll race you to the water. Last one in buys the beer, she said laughing, running to the surf line.

John followed quickly behind.

Reaching the sea just ahead of John, she turned and kicked up water, splashing him. 'I won,' she laughed.

John quickly reciprocated and soaked her. The splashing contest got more and more boisterous and they laughed together like carefree teenagers.

The pair spent time having fun, swimming and wading in and out of the surf.

'Right Mister, now it's time to see how good you are on the surfboard,' she said launching the board through the surf and expertly leaping on. 'I'll show you how to do it,' she added paddling out through the breakers.

John watched as she eventually turned, caught a wave, stood and expertly rode the wave in, zigzagging as she went.

'Bravo!' he clapped, as she leapt off the board next to him.

'Right, your turn,' she directed.

'You've got to be joking.'

'Well at least lie on it. It's good fun.'

John lay on the board and paddled out to where the waves were breaking.

Hesitantly he turned and caught a wave.

'Stand up,' she shouted.

Not to be out done, John stood up for a few seconds before being pitched off.

They laughed at their 'wipe out' failures on the surfboard as each one took it in turn to demonstrate their differing levels of prowess.

Finally exhausted by their exploits, they stumbled back to their bags and flopped down on the large beach towel covering the fine sand.

'That was brilliant fun,' she laughed, lying back and cradling her head. 'Do you know, we can watch the sunset from here too,' Laura observed.

'A seaside sunset, that would be nice,' John said. 'Not in my wildest dreams could I ever have imagined ending the workday like this in the salt sea air,' he grinned.

After a few minutes just gazing at the sky, Laura knelt up and towelled herself off. John couldn't help admiring her shapely figure enhanced by the myriad water droplets which glistened on her tanned skin.

Although he did a lot of outdoor running and hence exposed to some sunshine, John's sun starved English body was comparatively insipid in contrast to Laura's olive tan.

Satisfied that she was dry enough, Laura put on a short white tee shirt over her revealing one piece cossie. 'That's better,' she said. 'I was starting to feel a bit chilly.'

'Yes, likewise,' John admitted, pulling on a jumper that he extracted from his rucksack.

'I'm impressed. You did well on the board,' she complimented. 'You're obviously fit.'

'Yes, I used to go to the gym regularly. Underneath all this chest hair my six pack has gone a bit flabby, so I'll have to find another gym.'

'You won't have any problems finding one,' she advised him. 'There are plenty of gyms around here.'

As the beer flowed and the evening wore on, they felt totally relaxed in each other's company, and the conversation turned to their previous love lives.

Chapter Twenty-three

'At the risk of upsetting you again, do you mind if I ask how come a lovely girl like you has not been grabbed up by a dashing young man,' John asked hesitantly.

'No, it's Ok. I...is this a professional analysis session or am I getting this consultation for free?' she joked.

'Sorry, I find people's background's intriguing. No. Apologies, I shouldn't be asking intrusive questions. I should forget the day job,' he scolded himself.

'No, it's alright. I...came to Australia mainly because I fell in love with a married man in New Zealand. Although, at the time I didn't know he was married and he had kids too,' Laura revealed.

'Ouch!'

'When I did eventually find out, he told me that he was going to leave his wife. But after six months of false promises and agro, when his wife found out, I decided to walk away from the relationship and leave. I wasn't prepared to be his 'bit on the side'. So I left home. And the worst part was, I left my Mum and Dad.'

'Hell of a big decision.'

'Yes it was.'

'Why Australia?'

'I'd previously thought about coming here to Oz anyway, so made the leap and decided never to get involved with men ever again.'

'He obviously hurt you badly.'

'Yes, he did. He broke my heart. At one stage, I was suicidal,' Laura volunteered.

'I can understand that. I've seen many patients brought to their lowest ebb by deceitful partners,' John said, sympathetically.

'Anyway enough of me. Let me turn the tables on you. You know about me, what about you, starting a new life in a new land, alone?' Laura probed.

'Yes, I suppose I owe you that confidence. I think we are kindred spirits,' he observed. 'I..I...err, lost my childhood sweetheart to cancer.'

'Oh, I'm so sorry. I shouldn't have asked.'

'No, it's alright, it's good to talk about it, really.'

'If you're sure,' Laura said, feeling uncomfortable.

'Yes, it's Ok.. We had been friends at infant school and kept our relationship intact throughout our various schooling and university lives. We were planning to set up home together, when out of the blue she fell ill and was diagnosed with breast cancer. Sadly, none of the treatments worked and after a long illness, she died.'

'That must have been terrible for you?'

'Yes it was and even worse. I crashed the car rushing to get her to a treatment session.'

'How awful!'

'She was badly injured and that added to the trauma of her illness. Unfortunately, it was too much for her gentle heart and she passed away.'

'You must have been devastated?'

'Yes, I was. I couldn't live with myself, as you can imagine. It was my carelessness that probably accelerated her death.'

'Heavens!'

I was chronically depressed. But one of my Uni lecturers took me in hand and convinced me that I shouldn't blame myself and that I had to move on, as she would have wanted me to.'

A tear ran down his cheek.

So after I dragged myself through all my training, just like yourself, I decided that a new start in a new country was the best way out. We'd often dreamt of coming here to live anyway, so it seemed the right thing to do.'

Laura put a sympathetic arm around his shoulders and kissed him on the cheek. 'My turn to give you a kiss now,' she said softly.

John smiled and wiped away another tear.

'Anyway, enough of the doom and gloom, we're here on a lovely beach with wonderful company, let's have another beer,' he suggested.

''Good idea, she said reaching for another can. 'I'll stick to my cokes though,' she added. 'I've got to drive us back.'

'OK, but when I've got a car, I will pay you back by being your chauffeur,' he suggested.

'Bless you,' she smiled, cosying up to him.

'What are all those lights, the other side of the bay?' he asked, opening up another tinny.

'Well, we're looking towards North Harbour and that's the Grotto lighthouse flashing.'

John gave an alcoholic guffaw. 'There you go again with those strange names. Grotto makes me think of Grotty,' he laughed.

'Oh it makes me think of Santa's grotto,' she tittered. 'See what you can make of this then, we are opposite Dobroyd Point,' she added, waiting for him to make another drunken remark.

'No sorry, I can't make anything out of that name, he chortled. 'So what's those lights further round, there then?' he asked, pointing out a highly illuminated section.

'That might be Surfers Pavilion, where we went for that lovely meal,' she advised him.

'We must dine there again soon,' he said.

'I'll look forward to it,' she smiled.

They sat silently side by side, content in each other's company. They watched a magnificent sunset. As the sun dipped down below the horizon it left a signature in the clouds painting an ever changing kaleidoscope. The hues of fiery red, softened to heavenly pink before finally disappearing. The gentle lapping of the waves provided a soothing lullaby as the light show finally came to an end.

'Well I suppose we ought to go,' Laura said, half-heartedly.

'Yes, the temperature's dropping and we soon won't be able to see where we're going,' John said, standing.

Reluctantly they gathered all their stuff together and brought their picnic to a close.

After they had stowed the surfboard back on the car and as they put the other bits in the boot, their hands touched.

'Oh your hand is really cold. Come here and let me warm you up,' he said, gently turning her around to face him.

'Thank you for a lovely evening. It was a wonderful surprise and I truly enjoyed your perfect company,' he said, drawing her close. He paused, his heart hammering and looked into her eyes as if seeking permission to complete the manoeuvre.

'Yes, it's Ok to kiss me,' she encouraged lustily. 'No apologies necessary, this time.'

Chapter Twenty-four

The two policemen were sitting in their patrol car having a break after investigating a break-in.

'Did you see that documentary about those dodgy landlords?' Sergeant Jon Baldy asked his probationer constable colleague Barry Noland.

'No Sarge. When was that on?' the youngster asked, continuing to tuck into a large 'door step' tuna and sweetcorn sandwich.

'It was on early this week. It was my mate, the Investigative reporter, Sophie Mcbid?' the Sergeant revealed.

'Your mate? A TV reporter! How do you know her?' Constable Noland asked, impressed that his work colleague knew a celebrity.

'Shall we say, we've done a few mutually beneficial deals in the past,' the Sergeant explained.

'What was she investigating?'

'She was exposing landlords who offer free accommodation to financially cash strapped female lodgers in return for giving the dirty sods sexual favours.'

'Bleeding perverts. Makes my blood boil, taking advantage of young girls down on their luck,' the young Policeman seethed.

'Mind you, I wouldn't say no if Sophie wanted to investigate me,' the Sergeant beamed. 'She's a right Stunner.'

'Yeah, good work if you can get it,' the young Policeman smirked.

'Apparently the TV company had been contacted by several young women about being abused by their landlords,' the veteran officer continued.

'Why didn't they report it to us then?' Barry Noland pondered.

'They said that they didn't want to report it to the police for fear of being evicted,' the veteran Policeman explained.

'That doesn't make sense. Why go to the television company then? Surely it would make it worse for them with all that publicity?' the young Policeman reasoned.

'Money I expect. They'd obviously sussed out that the television company would pay money for a story like that,' the sergeant suggested. 'And as they're on low wages, 'any port in a storm'.

'What do you mean, 'any port in a storm'?'

'Sorry youngster. It means that they'd go anywhere to get help,' the sergeant clarified. 'Perhaps they felt protected from being evicted by making their plight publicly visible on the TV.'

'Poor sods, I suppose being financially vulnerable, they were ideal victims of these unscrupulous landlords.'

'The bottom line is that we all need to live in a place of safety,' the sergeant said sympathetically. 'And these lechers made it anything but that.'

'I guess the girls put up with it because it's better than being out on the streets,' the young PC suggested.

'Yeah, but I wouldn't like to think that my daughter was conned into that sort of mess,' the Sergeant said firmly. 'They must lose all self-respect to end up doing that. It's just another form of prostitution.'

'Surely they could just refuse to…you know, complete the bargain, if you know what I mean?' the young Policeman suggested naively.

'No, the crafty lechers get them to sign a legal document with the terms and conditions in small print. The small print, of course, defines their sexual responsibilities.'

'So what did good old Sophie do in the documentary to expose these guys?'

'She posed as a homeless waitress, wearing hidden cameras, and met several of these Landlords. She cleverly talked them into graphically explaining what they wanted her to do if she lodged there.'

'And did they tell her?'

'Yes. They hedged around the subject at first,' the Sergeant amplified. 'But she got them to explain in graphic details how they wanted her to fulfil their perverted fantasies. Of course the guys didn't know they were being set up.'

"Good for her,' the young policeman said enthusiastically. 'I can just imagine their shock and humiliation when she exposed them publicly on TV.'

'Although I did hear from some of our colleagues that she gave some bad publicity to a couple of guys who were totally innocent,' the older policeman added.

'Oh bummer. I expect the TV company had to issue an apology?' the young officer suggested.

'No, they refused. She claimed they were just collateral damage and insinuated that they were probably guilty about some other devious landlord scheme anyway.'

'With no proof? Oh that's naughty,' Barry observed.

'Yes I know for a fact that she's a hard bitch and a tough negotiator. She doesn't always play by the rules, that's for sure,' the sergeant revealed.

'Is there another episode soon?'

'No, not yet. But I believe she's currently preparing for another one.'

Suddenly, the police radio burst into life interrupting their conversation. *'Oscar one from Oscar base.'*

The young constable picked up the microphone. 'Oscar one. Go ahead.'

'Reports of protest groups causing problems by the sheltered housing complex. Please proceed immediately and give a Sit Rep.

'Sit Rep?' the youngster puzzled.

'Situation report,' the other explained.

'Roger. On our way. Oscar one, out.'

The PC switched on the blue lights as the sergeant 'gunned' the engine. The patrol car shot off in a squeal of tyre smoke heading for the disturbance.

Chapter Twenty-five

Within ten minutes of the radio call, the police car arrived at the site of the reported disturbance. The policemen were confronted by two groups of protestors noisily facing each other.

'Strewth, the young PC declared.

'No worries,' the Sergeant reassured him, bringing the car to a halt fifty yards from the melee. 'This is small. About twenty each side I would think. So long as they keep shouting at each other, we'll be Ok. But keep your eyes open for the lone agents who gets carried away. That's often when it turns nasty.'

'Ok,' the PC uttered, his mouth dry with fear.

'Let's see now,' the veteran Policeman said sizing up the protagonists. We've got one group, obviously they're the anti-mental health protesters with their posh placards.'

'What does that one say?' the young policeman said, straining his eyes to read the banners. *'Our Mental Health services are barbaric; Chemical Imprisonment is wrong. The Institute of torture; Professor Philips chief torturer.* 'Who's this Professor chappie?' the PC asked.

'He's the head honcho at the Institute, the Sergeant explained.

'Well they obviously don't like him.'

'No. I've had to investigate some damage to his car done by this lot of, so called, do-gooders.'

'And what are those on that poster? Is it prisoners?'

'I think it's supposed to be pictures of 'so say' patients in handcuffs,' the Sergeant suggested. 'It's supposed to indicate that the patients are chemically shackled, I think.'

'Yeah, compare that with the other lot's placards. Obviously hastily scribbled, misspelt banners from the social housing estate locals. Look *'Fritened for our kids safety' 'Nutters on the loose. Lock em up, Rope them,'* the young PC recounted.

'Yeah, you can see where the money is can't you?' the other acknowledged. 'But the toffs have got to be careful, a lot of these locals are regular troublemakers, just looking for a fight.'

'Oh crikey,' the young policeman said nervously.

'They often use the Institute patients as an excuse for starting bother,' the Sergeant explained. 'They justify their agro by saying that they are scared by the odd and erratic behaviour of the residents from the sheltered housing.'

'Mind you I've seen a few patients with er...with issues and they can be pretty scary,' the PC admitted.

'Thing is, irrespective of their views, the patients also have the right and freedom to roam in their own community. And we're here to protect their rights too,' the veteran policeman reminded him.

'So what you're saying is, there aren't any no-go areas here then?' the young PC summarised.

'No but there could be, if we allowed this sort of thing to carry on,' the sergeant explained, scanning the crowd again.

'There's some tough looking locals down there who seem to be pushing for a fight,' the PC observed. 'Glad that there doesn't appear to be any vulnerable patients down there at least.'

'Don't be fooled, they're not all innocent either. I've had to deal with some vicious patients too,' he informed his frightened colleague.

'Oh, have you?' the young Policeman managed to croak.

'I can understand why the locals might feel aggrieved,' the veteran Policeman said.

'Why?'

'Well the locals haven't got a lot to brighten their day. But when they see these bloody 'do gooders' come here in their posh clothes and fast cars, they get upset about being dictated to them about tolerance and understanding.'

'Well, perhaps they should be. What's the expression? Live and let live isn't it?'

'Live and let live! You should see where most of the locals live. Calling it basic squalor, is probably being too complimentary.'

'That bad?'

'Yeah. The only thing that brightens up the gloom of the estate comes from a few pocket lawns populated by malformed daisies, damaged dandelions and grey insipid clover.'

'Sounds attractive,' the PC said, sarcastically.

'Not to mention the persistent weeds that burst through the cracks in the unrepaired blanket of tarmac,' the Sergeant continued.

'Surely it can't be as bad as that?'

'Believe me, it is. The sunshine that occasionally manages to penetrate through the badly planned maisonettes, only lifts the atmosphere from gloom to less gloomy.'

'Poor sods.'

'Oh well, time for action.' The veteran Policeman said, gunning the engine. 'Get ready to jump out when I stop,' he directed. 'Here we go.'

The Sergeant revved up the engine and in a squeal of tyre smoke drove 'hell for leather' down the middle of the two opposing groups using his car as a barrier. The protesters hastily stepped out of the way, just avoiding being hit as he skidded to a halt.

'Phew, that was a bit close Sarge,' the young Policeman said, dry lipped, frightened at the prospect of leaving the safety of the patrol car to confront the unruly mob.

'You got to show them who's boss in riot situations. Act tough or be overwhelmed,' the veteran Policeman declared.

'If you say so,' the rookie said, fearfully eyeing the crowd of tough looking individuals.

'Radio in that we can probably deal with this lot, but if they've got a spare car, some backup might be helpful,' the Sergeant instructed.

'Sarge, they're all hard cases,' the young PC said, assessing the odds.

'Not as hard as the lignum vitae of my baton,' the older Policeman assured him. 'Just make the call, cobber.'

Barry made the radio call as directed. But was less pleased with the response, that there were no other vehicles available to help.

'So it's just us then?' the young Policeman said nervously.

"Yes. Watch me.' The Sergeant said, putting his cap on and stepping out of the car.

'RIGHT YOU LOT,' he shouted. 'I'LL GIVE YOU TWO MINUTES TO DISPERSE OR I SHALL BE ARRESTING THE LOT OF YOU. AND YOU'LL BE BEHIND BARS QUICKER THAN YOU KNOW IT.'

The shouting died down apart from a few yobs at the back of the crowd who were still looking for a fight.

'Don't take any notice of him,' one of the yobs instructed his compatriots. 'He can't arrest all of us.'

Meanwhile, nearby Marilyn had dragged Eddy outside their houses after hearing the police siren and had come to investigate.

'Come on Eddy, ' she said, excited at the prospect of a fight. 'If the yobs want a fight, they'll soon regret it,' Marilyn said, balling her fist.

'You know I don't like violence,' Eddy reminded her, attempting to drag her back towards his house. 'Let's go back in. Come on.'

'No not yet. Don't worry Eddy. I'll protect you,' she said, holding his hand. 'I've got a knife anyway,' she added producing a large kitchen knife from her pocket as they walked towards the source of the noise.

As they rounded a corner, unfortunately, the pair were spotted by a group of local rabble-rousers. Marilyn looked at the crowd of protesters and said 'Great. Punch up time.'

Eddy froze on the spot in fear.

'There! Look there's two of them,' a yob sporting a Mohican hair style, shouted. 'Let's get 'em.'

But before the group could move, the veteran Policeman, who had seen Eddy and Marilyn arrive, moved quickly towards them.

'Oh no you don't,' he said, standing in front of the yobs with his hand resting on his revolver. 'Now, back off, before you regret your actions.'

However, ignoring the Policeman's warning, one of the yobs dodged round the Sergeant and ran flat out at Eddy and Marilyn.

Taken by surprise, the Policeman was unable to stop him and the yob 'drop kicked' Eddy in the back as he was about to run away, knocking him to the ground.

Chapter Twenty-six

Marilyn quickly recovered from the surprise of the attack and immediately tackled the assailant before the Policeman could even respond.

Fortunately, the knife that she had been holding, was knocked out of her hand,

Not expecting the woman to fight back, the yob dropped his guard as he gloated at Eddy on the floor, but soon regretted his inattention.

Marilyn connected with a right hook to the yobs jaw, the likes of which any boxer would have been envious.

An angry red mist overcame the calming effect of her chemical shackles and her viciousness knew no bounds as she laid into him in a frenzy of punching. Under the torrent of blows the yob was knocked down, falling on his back.

Marilyn quickly seized the opportunity and straddled the prostrate yob and continued punching him mercilessly in the face while her opponent tried desperately to block the blows.

The Policeman watched as the pair grappled, biding his time, satisfied that the attacker was being punished 'urban jungle' style.

In the meantime, an apparently concerned woman broke away from the Anti-psychiatry protesters and rushed over to help the prostrate Eddy.

Sophie Mcbid recognised that Marilyn and Eddy were patients from the Institute by the grey tracksuits that they were wearing. Her good Samaritan act had an ulterior motive. She realised that it might give her the opportunity to befriend the pair and access inside information about the running of the institute from a patients point of view.

In spite of their nefarious financial dealings, the Police Sergeant didn't recognise Sophie, in her convincing disguise.

The television journalist was wearing a short black wig, which hid her long auburn hair; a pair of heavy framed spectacles and a mouthpiece giving her bulging front teeth that changed the shape of her mouth and face; cleverly applied makeup completed her alter ego.

Sophie had gone undercover, in pursuit of evidence for her investigations and embedded herself with the anti-psychiatry protesters for her proposed documentary.

But she needed to find out, first-hand, details about an alleged drug trial being run by the psychiatric hospital. And to obtain confirmation of the rumoured drug excesses and misuse. Hopefully these two patients would help her find the details that she needed.

Turning the prostrate Eddy over on to his back she quickly checked him out. 'That was a hell of a fall you had. Are you alright? Where does it hurt?' she asked earnestly.

'My...my...head,' Eddy uttered, sitting up and tentatively touching his forehead.

'Let me have a look,' she said examining his face. 'It's not bleeding but I think you will have a bump. Just rest awhile,' she said, moving around and laying him back down to cradle his head on her lap.

Mildly concussed and still woozy from the assault, Eddy saw his rescuer with diadems of light around her head, like a halo; her voice coming from a long way off, as if in a tunnel. Everything was happening around him in slow motion.

'Are you an angel?' he muttered, squinting at her.

'No. I'm just a concerned bystander trying to help you,' she replied.

'Well you look like an angel to me,' he said, before passing out.

In spite of continuing to batter Eddy's unfortunate assailant, out of the corner of her eye Marilyn was aware of Eddy's condition.

She didn't like what she saw. Another woman was touching Eddy.

Further angered by the stranger interfering with her man, her hackles rose more and resulted in her giving the yob an even more severe beating.

Finally, the Sergeant decided that Marilyn had delivered enough punishment to the now bleeding and defenceless yob, so he intervened at last.

'Right you two. Pack it up now,' he ordered, grabbing hold of Marilyn's arm as she was just about to deliver another right hook.

Using all his strength, he forcibly dragged her off the troublemaker.

As soon as Marilyn was off him, the yob ran off, leaving a blood trail from his facial injuries.

'Don't you come back round here again,' she shouted. 'Or I'll finish you off next time.'

'Right that will do,' the Policeman said calmly, letting her go.

Marilyn rushed to Eddy and glared at Sophie who was still cradling his head in her lap.

'I'll do that now,' she said grabbing hold of her unconscious friend and hugging him. 'Oh Eddy, are you alright?' Marilyn said anxiously.

'I think he's just a bit shocked,' Sophie offered. 'You were very brave tackling that man.'

'I was very very, angry,' Marilyn panted. 'If I hadn't dropped that knife I would have stabbed him and stabbed him, until he was dead,' she said, becoming frighteningly animated.

'And then you would have been in real trouble,' the Policeman said, overhearing the conversation.

'I don't care. He hurt my Eddy. He better not come back here again,' she ranted angrily, her hands shaking as adrenalin still charged through her body.

'Is he alright?' the Sergeant asked Sophie.

'Yes, I think so. He's not bleeding as far as I can see, but he'll have a nice bump on his head and possibly a black eye by morning.' she replied, pleased that the Policeman still didn't recognise her under the elaborate disguise.

'Ok, I'll leave you with him, while I help my colleague to disperse the crowd,' he said, leaving the trio.

'Are you from the sheltered houses too?' Sophie asked Marilyn, already knowing the answer from their Institute's tracksuit uniform.

'Yes. We both are. But those people who come here are horrible to us.' Marilyn revealed.

'Interesting! Hi, I'm Sheila,' she lied, offering her hand. ' What's your name?'

Marilyn looked at the proffered hand suspiciously but didn't understand the gesture and ignored it. Sophie dropped her hand.

'My name is Marilyn,' she replied.

'And I assume this is Eddy?'

'Yes, he is my friend.'

'Are you married?'

'Oh no. Not married,' Marilyn tittered at the suggestion. 'Not married,' she repeated, smiling at the thought.

Eddy stirred. 'Oh my head!' he groaned, sitting up, rubbing his forehead. 'Has that man gone? he asked fearfully, quickly looking around.

'Yes the horrible man has gone,' Marilyn confirmed.

'And you're Ok Eddy.' Sophie said quietly. 'You're not bleeding. Just give yourself a bit of time to clear your head. Marilyn, do you get a lot of problems from the residents round here?'

'Yes,' Marilyn confirmed. 'But I fight them when I have to.'

'Interesting. Well I'm going to be around here for some time. Eddy, perhaps we could all meet for a coffee one day?' she suggested.

'Yes that would be nice,' Eddy agreed.

Marilyn was clearly uncomfortable with Sophie's suggestion. She stood up and grabbed Eddy's hand and pulled him to his feet, away from Sophie. 'Come on Eddy. We got to go.'

'Why?'

Because we have to,' she said, jealously aware of Sophie's developing closeness to her friend.

'Ok.'

'I'll be in touch,' Sophie called to the departing pair. 'Yes, indeed,' she smirked. 'I have a way in.'

As the last of the crowd disappeared, it was only the two Policeman left.

'Did you see that Marilyn with that knife, Jon?'

'Yes, and she threatened to stab him too,' the PC replied. 'She's a nasty piece of work that one.'

'Yes, she is. I have my suspicions whether she had anything to do with that Digger Lucas murder,' the Sergeant pondered. 'Hopefully, the fingerprints on the knife should tell the tale.'

'Any ideas when they're likely to come back?'

'No. But I hope it's before anyone else ends up the same way.'

Chapter Twenty-seven

The following day Marilyn barged into Eddy's house to find Eddy on the settee, still in his night clothes, half asleep.

'Why aren't you dressed Eddy?' she demanded.

'I didn't sleep well. I keep thinking about the man coming back and hitting me again.'

'No, you're safe here. That man won't do that again, I'll protect you,' Marilyn reassured him.

'And my head and back hurts too.'

'It looks like you've got a black eye and there's a lump on your forehead. Does it hurt?' she said, studying his face.

'Just a bit,' he said, gingerly touching the bump.

'It'll be fine,' she said dismissively. 'I've got bruised knuckles where I beat the guy up. You could at least say thank you.'

'Thank you? Thank you for what?'

'Rescuing you from that yob.'

'Oh yes. Thank you very much. I hope your knuckles get better soon,' he said awkwardly.

'I expect they will. They usually do after I've been fighting.' Marilyn said glibly.

'But what if you're not around if he comes here?' Eddy said fearfully.

'I'll be,' she said, sitting next to him and hugging him. 'I'm not going away.'

'That lady was nice wasn't she?' Eddy said, sitting up.

'What lady?' Marilyn glowered.

'The one that looked like an angel after that man knocked me down,' he explained.

'Well she isn't. And I don't want her coming round here or seeing you again,' Marilyn ranted.

'No, Ok. If you say so.'

'I do. And if she tries…I'll…I'll…' Marilyn started to say, clenching her fists.

Eddy interrupted her. 'I had that weird dream again last night. I keep having dreams. 'They wake me up,' he moaned.

'What dream?'

'I was a kid and I went into a big shop with my Dad to buy a train set and suddenly the lights dimmed and it became cold. And I grabbed for my Dad's hand but when I turned around he had disappeared. I looked everywhere for him but I couldn't find him and then I was chased by horrible toys and attacked by an emu and….

'Oh that nightmare,' Marilyn said dismissively. 'I don't see my parents either. Not anymore…after the fire,' Marilyn volunteered.

But Eddy wasn't listening, he was in a world of his own. 'When I see Doctor John's face it makes me feel sad…' Eddy recounted. 'And sometimes a spooky voice says you'll make a good doctor, someday…someday…someday. Like I'm in an echo chamber. But then another voice says, you lost a patient…lost a patient. But, I don't know why. It's very spooky.' Eddy relayed.

'Yeah I have strange dreams too,' Marilyn added. I dream that I can do back flips. But when I try, I always end up flat on my back instead. Sometimes I've got to go to casualty because I've really hurt my back.'

'Dreams are strange things, aren't they?' he said standing up and going into the bathroom and standing in the shower.

'Eddy what are you doing?'

'I'm going to have a shower.'

'Don't you normally take your clothes off first?' Marilyn suggested. 'And don't forget to close the bathroom door.'

'Oh! Oh yeah. That's right I do don't I?' he said closing the door. 'I'm just taking my clothes off now and I'm turning the shower on,' he announced.

'You don't need to give me a running commentary. Just have your shower,' she instructed.

'Oh, OK.'

'I think the Professor wants to check our progress today on the trial,' Marilyn shouted over the noise of the shower.

'Well I took my pills early this morning and I've got to have another one in a minute,' Eddy revealed. 'But I don't feel right. My heads full of cotton wool.'

'No that's not right, I don't think you should feel like that,' Marilyn said. 'That's why I think someone should check you over. Perhaps it was the bang on the head?'

'Ok Marilyn,' Eddy agreed…'Whatever you say.'

'Perhaps Doctor John will do it. When did you say he was going to see you again?'

'I think that it's tomorrow,' Eddy said towelling himself off and walking out of the bathroom naked.

'Eddy, put some clothes on. I don't want to see your willy,' Marilyn barked and averted her eyes.

Chapter Twenty-eight

It was a week after Eddy's first session with John, that he arrived on time outside the consulting room door for his appointment. He knocked gently.

'Come on in Eddy,' the psychiatrist invited.

Eddy entered, less apprehensive than on the previous occasion.

'Hello Eddy, thanks for coming. How are you? Oh I can see that you have been in the wars,' John observed spotting Eddy's black eye.

'The wars! What do you mean?' Eddy puzzled. 'I haven't been to war.'

'Sorry, it's an expression that people sometime use when someone has been hurt and have injuries.'

'Oh, I see...'

'Tell me what happened.'

'I was hurt by a nasty man yesterday. It was horrible,' Eddy explained, feeling the bump on his forehead.

'I'm sorry to hear that,' John sympathised. 'Yes, I heard about the demonstration and it sounds like you were in the wrong place at the wrong time. Are you ok though?'

'I've a bump on my head and a black eye. And I feel like I've got cotton wool in my brain and I had a nightmare,' Eddy gushed, without pausing for breath.

'A nightmare! That's interesting. Can you remember what it was about?'

'I...I...keep hearing voices and see faces,' Eddy revealed, but withheld that it was actually John's face that was haunting him. Instead he explained briefly about the dream.

'I dreamed that I was left by my Dad in a toy shop and when I wanted him to buy me a train set, he disappeared, I couldn't find them.'

'Interesting! Ok we'll try and find out during the session what happened shall we?.

'Ok.'

'Did you have any problems after our session last week?' John asked, trying to tease more information out from Eddy.

'No, I don't think so.'

'Right, if you'd like to sit on the couch for me, please,' the psychiatrist invited.

Within a few moments, John put Eddy back into a hypnotic state, suitably wired up with the EEG cap and started a series of questions. Rechecking that Eddy's answers from the first session correlated with todays.

'Remember you are an observer watching Eddy. What does he remember about coming to Australia?'

'He was very little. It was on a big ship and he was excited.'

'Who was with him?'

'His Dad and his new wife Beverley, his step-mother.'

'That's good. Now where was Eddy before he came to this hospital in Manly?' John prompted.

Eddy became restless.

'Was Eddy still happy with his family life?'

'No. All the happiness went away. Instead there was black sorrow,' Eddy relayed.

John was surprised at the sudden depressing tone in Eddy's voice as he relayed the story. 'What happened to him?'.

'Foster parents. Horrible, Orphanage, Mental Asylums. He felt so alone. Nobody loved him.

'Why was he in the orphanage?' John probed, confused.

'No parents.'

'Why, what happened to his parents?'

And then Eddy's alpha wave pattern became frantic. He thrashed about on the couch as if trying to ward something off.

'I can't. I don't want to say. It must never be talked about.' Eddy said hysterically. 'No I mustn't. I can't. It is too painful.'

'Ok Eddy, just take your time and relax again. Let those bad thoughts go. Relax…relax,' John intoned.

Eddy relaxed on the couch. The frantic trace on the monitor slowed and eventually flattened.

'Let's go to when he first came here under this hospital's care. Was he happy then?'

'Yes. He wasn't alone anymore. He met Marilyn; She is very brave, she stood up for him; she has laughing brown eyes. He likes her very much.' Eddy revealed.

'And what about the Professor ?

'He gave him stuff for his nightmares.'

'Were they bad nightmares?'

'Yes.'

'Can he remember anything about them?'

There was a pause while Eddy obviously struggled with something in his memory.

'No. He doesn't want to remember. They make him feel so bad,' Eddy uttered starting to twist and turn again. The monitor reflecting his inner turmoil.

'But did the Professors pills help him?'

'Yes.'

'OK Eddy, I think we've done enough for today. Take your time to come back. Just relax. There is no rush.

Eddy slowly slipped out of the trance.

'Thank you Eddy for today.'

'Did you find anything to help me in the toy shop?'

'No not yet. But it will only be a matter of time before I do. Don't worry.'

After Eddy had fully recovered, John showed him out.

'I need to do a bit more research into Eddy's background, so that I can fire off more appropriate trigger questions,' he decided. 'Irrespective of what the Professor was saying about not using hypnotherapy, I need to see Eddy's records.

'And I wonder if that will reveal the question of why he dreams about being deserted. Clearly he had two parents over here. So what happened to them? Perhaps that's what I need to find out'

Chapter Twenty-nine

Later that morning, John bumped in to the Professor.

'I suppose that against my advice you have started your hypnotherapy sessions with Eddy?' the Professor said brusquely.

'Yes, I...I...err thought it would help unravel his psychological tensions.'

'And has it?'

'Well, I've only had a couple of sessions with him so far, but it's like getting blood out of a stone. Mentally, he keeps blocking me out. There's something about his father that goes deep into his subconscious that he doesn't want to relive.' John explained, ignoring the Professor's negativity.

'What do you mean?' the Professor asked suspiciously.

'When I took him back to the time he came to Australia, he was quite open. Then when I probed a bit more, specifically talking about his father, he clammed up.'

'I'm not a bit surprised. I think you are wasting your time. I've seen these 'so called' encouraging sessions before. In the end however, it all goes wrong. These mental blockages are there for a specific reason.'

'Could you elucidate,' John queried.

'Yes of course. It's the brains way of protecting itself against further trauma,' the Professor explained. 'When we interfere by probing too deeply, we take away it's natural protective barrier.'

'That's a new one on me,' John observed, sceptically.

'The danger is, that when we do that, we leave the patient in a more psychologically vulnerable condition than when we started,' the Professor explained.

'Well, let's hope not,' John said, although secretly wondering if the Professor had a point. Perhaps removing Eddy's protective barrier would indeed undermine his overall mental health.

'Anyway, I hope that you're wrong,' John said resolutely. 'Time alone will tell. In the meantime can you tell me where I can find Eddy's medical records?'

'Why do you want to see those?' the Professor asked suspiciously.

'So that I can target my questioning better.'

'Well I...I'm not sure. The last time I tried to find them, they were missing perhaps misfiled,' he lied. 'I'll get someone to check for you,' he volunteered.

'No, it's Ok, I'll get Laura to hunt them down for me, thanks,' John added quickly.

'Well, mark what I've said. Don't waste your time on dead ends,' the Professor said firmly. 'There's lots to be done here with other patients as well as taking over from me.'

'Yes, I'll make sure that looking after Eddy doesn't compromise anything else. Thank you anyway,' John said stiffly, and left.

The Professor watched him leave and when John was out of sight he headed straight to the records office.

As he entered reception he was pleased to see that Laura was not at her desk. He quickly made his way past it and entered the ground floor record office. In case Laura was already in there, he went warily to the suite of document file drums.

Relieved that she wasn't there, he manually turned the appropriate drum round until he found Eddy's file, exactly where it should be. Correctly filed, as he'd expect.

Checking that he was not going to be disturbed, the Professor opened Eddy's file and quickly removed a sheet recording the data from his experimental trial.

'Nobody else needs to see that,' he thought, as he quickly pocketed the incriminating sheet.

He returned Eddy's file back, out of order where he'd found it, to give credence to his 'misfiled' story.

He hurriedly left the records room, just as Laura returned with John in tow.

'Oh I see you've called for assistance in your quest,' the Professor said as he rushed past them.

'Yes. Laura said she will track it down for me. I'm sure she'll find it,' John replied optimistically.

The pair entered the records office and John closed the door.

'So what did you want?'

'Eddy Jones records, please.'

'It'll cost you,' Laura said salaciously.

'What did you have in mind,' he smiled.

'A kiss for starters,' Laura purred, moving closer.

Checking that no one arriving in reception could see them, John put his arms around her waist and pulled her to him.

'What have I done to deserve this?' he asked thickly.

'Just thanking you for that lovely evening we shared.', Laura said meekly.

'What if someone comes in?'

'Then we'll have to be quick,' she said, gently planting her lips on his.

'You are terrible young lady,' he cooed, returning her lingering kiss.

'Anyway, to business,' she said suddenly, turning away from him. 'Whose file did you say you wanted?' Laura asked, her head in a spin from the sudden intimacy.

'Yours to start off,' he said, hugging her from behind and nuzzling her neck.

'Someone might come in,' she warned mildly.

'Possible discovery makes it even more exciting. What can a man do against a ladies wiles,' he groaned letting her go. 'It's Eddy Jones. I'm trying to exorcise his demons through hypnotherapy, but he's resisting at the moment and I need to get some more background material to target my questioning.'

'Ok, lets' have a look shall we?'

Laura went straight to the section of the large circular document drum that the records were under. 'J for Jones? you said?'

'Yes.'

'Oh, you're in luck. J is right on top,' she said shuffling the files. 'No it's not where it should be. Let's, just…have a look,' she said checking. 'Ah here we are. It was misfiled a few records away.'

'Oh thank you very much. I'll repay you later,' he smiled, giving her another peck.

'I hope so,' she teased. 'I'll record that the file is with you then. In the unlikely event that anyone else needs it, they'll know where to go.'

The pair parted company and John made his way back to his office, quite excited that he was going to be able to investigate Eddy's background.

Chapter Thirty

John placed Eddy's file on his desk and made himself a coffee.

Cup in hand he opened the dog eared folder.

As he studied the documentation he was disappointed to discover that it was all a bit sketchy. Not a lot of detail in the early years of Eddy's treatment either. And surprisingly, it seemed to end prematurely.

'No current data! Surely the Professor or my predecessor would have been recording his progress or treatment? Odd!' John thought.

He carried on leafing through the file looking for the basic information which should have been recorded right at the beginning of his healthcare, when Eddy first started receiving treatment.

'It looks like he was only ten when he started having treatment for mental health issues. Poor kid.

No parents recorded here either!' he puzzled, rescanning the document. 'That's odd. Eddy told me that he came over to Australia with Father and Stepmother. So why have they suddenly vanished?

Perhaps it's just an admin error! Alternatively, did something catastrophic happen to his parents. Was Eddy orphaned? Judging by his reactions to my questions, I fear the latter. So I wonder what the story is there then? Perhaps that's the reason for his nightmares,' John mused.

'Well whatever it was, it appeared to happen over a short period of time. The poor lad ended up being put into care and then, for some reason, pitched into the Mental Health system.

It all points to some tragic event occurring. If that's the case then clearly, the loss of Eddy's stable base, his home, and family would give him some form of childhood bereavement.

If my theory is right, that form of traumatic stress would manifest itself as the likely cause of his mental issues. Probably institutionalising him and using the blunt instrument of unsophisticated medication wouldn't have helped either.'

Leafing through the file John also found some sketchy notes from the Social Care department.

'Edward is a quiet, nicely spoken, intelligent boy. Who keeps himself to himself and consequently doesn't have any friends. He has little interaction with the adults in the foster home.

'So, it appears that he was sent to a foster home first, where suddenly the quiet intelligent little boy became *'moody with violent outbursts'*. So what's going on there?' John wondered.

There are several sessions of *'appropriate physical discipline'* recorded too. Presumably, that's code for 'the belt. Looks like the foster parents were disciplinarians and consequently gave him a good hiding for his angry outbursts.

Then Eddy was sent into an orphanage. I guess when this brutal regime in the foster home failed to bring any improvements they gave up on him.

Poor kid, it looks like the orphanage proved to be an even worse disaster for him. It appears that Eddy was bullied here. Yes here's some records of *bruising, split lips and black eyes*. Oh dear, one disaster after another.

The stress must have been awful for the kid. Like a lot of these orphanages, I bet no-one gave him any emotional support for whatever trauma he had experienced.

I can just imagine that 'inside' his intelligent little mind, he was still raging against his cruel fate.'

And then John spotted a record of Eddy's medical treatment which confirmed his analysis.

'Oh yes, here we go, the good old fallback; when all else fails stick them under a 'medical health scheme' and heavily tranquilise them to calm them down. Totally misdiagnosed. Poor youngster.'

John's blood boiled at the injustice of 'the system' that had robbed Eddy of a normal development into adulthood.

'They just couldn't be bothered with him,' he ranted to himself. 'And of course they 'proved' their case because now medically suppressed I suppose he was no trouble to anyone, anymore.

The worse thing is that sadly, nothing was done to treat the original cause of Eddy's condition, his depression from losing his stable base, his family.'

Leafing through the records the story showed that as he grew from youngster, through his teens to adulthood in this suppressed state, he still fought against his medication and became occasionally problematic, including obsessing about elements of the medical profession.

'Well I witnessed that on the ferry coming here on day one,' John said to himself.

'What's this? Eddy had to be cautioned several times for posing as a doctor or ambulance worker. How peculiar!'

At the back of the file, John found a small article cut out from a newspaper. It was badly faded, the newsprint very difficult to read.

'The headline read **Dramatic rescue**

Tourist Doctor Justin Jones and son Eddy(10) were dramatically rescued by fireman after their car was involved in a crash on a forest track. The boy was alone for some time with his injured father until they were eventually rescued. Doctor Jones was seriously hurt in the collision. Father and son were airlifted out and taken to hospital.

'Ah ha, at last. Pity I can't read the rest. However. this is obviously the key to his problems,' he beamed. 'But it doesn't say whether his father died and there's no mention of his step mother being involved in the accident either. So what happened to them? The mystery deepens.'

Chapter Thirty-one

'Well, were Eddy's records any use?' Laura asked, as she delivered John's post later.

'Yes they were, thanks. It looks like Eddy has had a bit of a tough life and didn't experience a normal childhood.'

'What do you mean, a normal childhood?'

'He's been fostered, stuck in an orphanage and finally got put in to a mental health 'merry-go-round.'

'Why was that?' Laura quizzed.

'I couldn't understand why until I found a small newspaper cutting at the back of the file. Eddy was apparently involved in a car accident with his father when he was only ten. Doctor Jones was reported to be seriously injured but it doesn't say whether Eddy sustained any injuries.

Apparently Eddy was alone with his father before some fire fighters rescued them from a forest track.'

'Poor kid. That must have been terrible for him. No wonder he is like he is, after being involved in that sort of trauma.'

'Yes he obviously suffered from some form of post-traumatic stress. I wonder! Do you think that we can find some more about the actual incident?' John mused.

'How will that help?' Laura asked.

'If I can get him to actually physically revisit the place of this trauma, I'm sure that I can talk him through addressing the fear of the ghosts in his mind,' John explained.

'Interesting, but how will you achieve that?'

'Firstly, we need to know the precise location of the accident site,' John suggested.

'That's not going to be easy,' Laura pointed out. 'Judging by Eddy's age at the time of the accident. What was he, ten?'

'Yes, and he's thirty five now,' John added.

'Heavens, it happened twenty five years ago.' Laura observed.

'Yes. Not going to be easy,' John agreed.

'Well in that case, the only place to look would be newspaper archives,' Laura suggested. 'Does that cutting show what newspaper it's from?'

'No,' John said, checking the frail bit of newsprint. 'But it's got a date on it though,' he informed her, scrutinising the cutting.

'Well I suppose that's a start. Without it we'd be on an impossible mission. As it is, it's going to be a massive undertaking trying to search all the newspaper archives in Australia anyway. Without a date, it would be completely impossible.' Laura observed.

'Well at least we know it was in a forest somewhere,' John said, unhelpfully.

'Brilliant observation,' she said, sarcastically. 'There are an awful lot of forests in New South Wales let alone in the Australian continent.'

'Ok, something else to consider. Eddy was telling me that he loved fishing with his father. At which, in spite of his trance state, he became agitated.'

'That's pretty slim evidence to go on though. So what have we got? A date; a forest, a forest with fishing nearby. Could be anywhere,' she summarised pessimistically.

'As you have a lot of local knowledge about the Australian geography and likely newspapers of the area, would you mind investigating for me?' he asked tentatively.

'Are you sure that this will help Eddy?' she queried. 'It's going to be an awful lot of work.'

'Yes, I'm certain,' he said optimistically. 'I would hope that we can improve Eddy's future by revisiting his past. It's a proven technique,' he reassured her. And it's becoming more accepted by the psychiatric world.'

'Becoming?'

'Yes. It's still in it's infancy as a technique,' John admitted.

'Ok, I'll do my best. But don't hold your breath. It's likely to take some time.'

'Thank you, I knew I could rely on you. Oh one thing that might help. Eddy told me that his father was a Doctor and they lived in Sydney. I'm assuming that he could have been a GP,' he suggested.

'Yes, but equally he could have been a hospital doctor too,' Laura pointed out.

'Let's try the GP route to start off with,' John proposed.

'Ok, whatever you wish. GPs of twenty five years ago, it is then.' Laura agreed.

'I suppose, if we could track him down to a practice, that would be a good start.'

'I agree and even better if any of his former colleagues are still alive,' Laura added.

'Perhaps they could provide some more details about the accident and Eddy's background?' John suggested, optimistically.

'Yes, I suppose that's another possible source,' Laura agreed. 'Did Eddy say whereabouts in Sydney his father was practising?'

'No, sorry. But his name was Justin Jones'

'Ok, I'll see what I can do.'

'Thanks. Good luck,' John smiled.

'Perhaps the Professor could also fill in some gaps?' Laura suggested.

'Worth a try too, I guess. But don't mention my hypnotherapy sessions. We are at opposing views on Eddy's treatment regime.'

Chapter Thirty-two

Sophie wasted no time in 'cosying up' to Eddy. Here was her way in to finding out the 'inner secrets' of the Institute, she thought.

It took her a few visits loitering around the sheltered housing area wearing her disguise before she 'accidently' bumped into Eddy. She found him sat on the bench alone.

'Hello Eddy, how are you now?'

'Oh hello...ummm...Sorry, I...I don't remember your name,' he apologised.

'You might not know it anyway, it's Sheila,' she lied.

'I am fine thank you. Umm. Sheila. Thank you for looking after me when that man hit me and knocked me down.'

'That's Ok. I'm glad that you are OK. I was very concerned,' she lied. 'I wonder if you would like to have a coffee with me?'

'Coffee! with you? I'd love to,' Eddy gushed, excited that this pretty woman would take the time to even speak to him, let alone take him for a drink.

'There's a café round the corner,' she smiled. 'We could go there.'

'Oh that's very kind of you. ...Oh, but I haven't got any money,' he suddenly remembered, patting the empty pockets of his tracksuit bottoms.

'It's Ok. I'll pay,' she volunteered. 'I'll claim it on my expenses anyway,' she thought.

Sophie led the pair to the café while Eddy trotted behind her to keep up with her business like purposeful walk.

'How long have you been in your new house Eddy?' she asked, over her shoulder.

'I don't know. When they were built, I think,' Eddy puffed, increasing his pace. 'We were specially selected.'

'You must have been very special then?' she suggested.

'Special! Yes we must have been special because we were the first to move in,' he agreed, smiling.

'Well you certainly live up to the special label,' Sophie thought cruelly.

'Eh, eh, eh. It was very exciting moving there from living in a hospital all the time,' he volunteered, excitedly.

'I bet it was,' she thought, visualising the chaos of seeing former 'prisoners' of the asylums testing their freedom for the first time.

'But we were all scared,' he said dramatically.

'Scared! Why?'

'Because we then had to do things for ourselves,' he revealed, miserably.

'What do you mean, do things for yourselves? she puzzled.

'Well you know, like making the bed, cooking our food and stuff,' he explained.

'Didn't they give you any help?' Sophie queried, immediately switching her brain into reporting mode, imagining possible headlines; *'Mental Health Shame; Patients Dumped with no help; De-institutionalised, left to fend for themselves'*.

'No, they didn't' Eddy shook his head. Feeling buoyed up that she was happy to talk to him and that he was telling her what he thought she wanted to hear.

Eddy however, conveniently forgot that the Institute had actually provided 'handholding' for them all for two weeks and were still currently closely monitoring them.

Eventually the pair arrived at the busy café. Eddy caught his breath, pleased that the route-march was over. Apprehensively he followed her in, expecting to be shouted at by the owner and told to get out like on previous occasions.

But to his surprise nothing happened. He followed closely behind Sophie, ostrich like, his eyes averted, hoping that no one would see him.

Sophie chose a table near the window and sat down; Eddy quickly sat down opposite her.

A waitress was immediately by their side. Eddy looked away, expecting to be admonished for being there.

However, much to his surprise, she simply asked Sophie, 'Can I get you something?'

Eddy relaxed. Perhaps Sophie was his guardian angel after all and while he was with her everything was going to be OK.

'What would you like Eddy?' Sophie asked.

'Could I have some chocolate, please?'

'Yes certainly,' the waitress confirmed. 'And you Madam?'

'A cup of black coffee, please.'

'Certainly.'

The waitress left to get the order.

'So how long have you been having treatment?' Sophie probed.

'Treatment? What do you mean?' Eddy asked, puzzled.

'Well how long were you with the hospital before you came here?'

'Oh, ages. I don't know,' he said dismissively.

'Do you take tablets to help you?' she probed.

'Yes. The Professor gives us special pills to help us feel better. We are special. We are on a trial,' he revealed.

'A trial! Really?' Sophie's ears pricked up. 'And is that all of you?'

'No, only some of us. The special ones who live in the block.'

'I see. And do the pills make you feel well?' she probed.

'Well yes, but...umm, but some people have been poorly and gone to a special place. That's sad isn't it?'

'Very sad,' she said, trying to sound sincere, but inwardly feeling smug that already she had a route in to revealing a scandal.

The waitress brought their order and Sophie dug into her purse and paid the bill but without a tip.

'I'd like a receipt,' she demanded.

'Yes, no worries,' the waitress said, giving her the bill.

Sophie was feeling smug that the small bribe of taking Eddy for a drink should already be so rewarding to her investigations.

'So, where's this special place that the others were going to?' she asked casually.

'I don't know. But some of them were our friends. And there was one nasty person who got stabbed.'

Sophie tensed at the mention of the stabbing, and subconsciously rubbed her arm.

'I didn't want them to go there, Eddy said quietly.'
'We can't see them anymore.'

'No that's quite sad isn't it? She said, trying to sound sympathetic. 'How many people have gone to this special place, Eddy?' she probed.

'Let me think. Mmm, there was Digger…umm; Peter and…umm; Oh Mathew, too.'

'Three people?' she checked.

'Yes.'

'That ties up with what the Sergeant had fed her,' she thought. 'The special place, obviously Eddy didn't know was the morgue.'

'And do you think they were all taking the special tablets that the Professor was giving them?' Sophie summarised.

'Yes. We all are.'

'So you are taking the tablets too Eddy. Is that right?'

'Ummm…Yes. But anyway, the new Doctor is treating me now. So I won't be taking them anymore.'

'A new doctor! What's his name?'

'Doctor John,' Eddy relayed innocently.

'Doctor John! Do you know his last name?

'It begins with a M…Mmm…'

'Masters?'

'Masters. Yes that's right,' he told her, pleased with himself.

'Sophie smiled, which made Eddy feel very happy.

'Is this new Doctor, giving you tablets as well?'

'No. He is using umm. hyp…hyp…I can't remember the word,' Eddy blustered.

'Hypnotherapy?' she suggested.

'Yes, that's right. Hypno thingamee,' he confirmed. 'But he's promised he won't turn me in to a chicken.'

Sophie laughed. 'A chicken! What do you mean not turning you into a chicken?' she puzzled.

'Only Marilyn said that she saw a hyp…a hypno person at the fair and he turned the people into chickens and they laid eggs.'

'Really,' she smirked.

'So how is he actually treating you?'

'On the couch with a hat of many coloured wires,' Eddy explained, gesturing by putting an imaginary hat on his head.

'A what?' she asked surprised.

Suddenly Eddy stood up; his eyes rolled into the back of his head.

'Eddy, Eddy are you Ok?' Sophie asked. Are you alright?' she repeated concerned.

No reply.

Chapter Thirty-three

Suddenly Eddy sprung to life. His hysterical laugh filled the cafe...the clink of cutlery and conversation, immediately stopped. Anxiously people turned to see what was going on.

Sophie's face had taken on a new colour. It was covered in a brown liquid. It dripped off her eyebrows, like brown stalactites.

With shock and disbelief etched on her face, her scream came a split second after his hysterical laugh.

Eddy beamed, he thought she resembled a melting chocolate hedgehog.

'That was clever, Sheila how did you do that ?' Eddy asked innocently, his eyes filled with laughter tears.

'You bloody maniac. What the hell do you think you're doing?' she screeched.

'What do you mean. I didn't do anything,' Eddy said, innocently.

'Yes you did. You frigging idiot. You just threw your drink in my face.'

'I never.....' he said, confused. 'It wasn't me.'

People rushed to her side.

'Are you alright Miss? Quick grab him before he does anything else to her,' someone shouted. 'He's one of those nutters from the sheltered housing.'

Hands grabbed Eddy's arms.

'Get off me,' Eddy said, trying to shrug off the restraining hands. 'I didn't do anything. I was just talking to her and...suddenly she had a brown face.'

'You should get to the hospital. Your face, might be scolded,' a woman customer suggested.

'Who did it Sheila? Tell me and I'll...I'll get Marilyn to hit them...I won't let them do it again. She'll protect you, like she protects me.'

'Don't come that with me, Eddy. You know very well who. It was you...you did it....it was you... you silly sod...what did you want to do that for ?' Sophie screeched.

'I never...' Eddy pleaded, feeling deeply hurt by the accusation. 'I didn't do anything.'

'Then why are you holding your empty cup like that?' she demanded, wiping her face gently with a paper serviette, conscious of possible damage to the heavy makeup of her disguise.

Eddy looked at his hand holding the empty cup and felt sad.

Sophie stood up, arms outstretched in dismay, looking down at her stained tea shirt and concerned that her disguise might be compromised.

'Look at this ...it's ruined...you stupid idiot,' she seethed.

'I would never do anything to hurt you Sheila.'

'Then who the bloody hell was it ?.....I bet it's that medication that you are on,' she suggested.

'Yes, it's the tablets of course...but...but'

'Are you still taking them?' she demanded, as she continued gently wiping her face and chest.'

'Yes,' Eddy said meekly. 'Although they make me feel weird. The Professor said I must take them for the trial.'

'Trial? Oh yes, the trial.' Despite the mess on her clothes, Sophie's journalistic curiosity was heightened by his mention of the trial.

'My friends and me are taking part in an important trial,' Eddy reiterated.

'Yes, so you've already said,' she reminded him, smiling to herself. 'If this is what I have to put up with for the sake of getting good data for my documentary. Then it's a small price to pay,' she reassured herself.

Eddy watched her wiping herself down, crestfallen at what he had done. Fearing his new friendship was about to be ended before it had really began.

But Sophie was already dreaming of a possible TV award and reassuring herself that she was right to befriend him. 'It will be worthwhile putting up with a bit of his nonsense in the end,' she thought.

The man who grabbed Eddy, started leading him out of the cafe. 'Come on my lad, it's time you weren't here.'

Annoyed at being manhandled, Eddy tried to disconnect himself from the man. 'Leave me alone. Get off me...'he demanded, desperately trying to break the handhold.

'It's Ok,. Don't hassle him.' Sophie said quietly. 'He'll only get upset...and who knows what he'll do next.'

'Ok,' the man said, letting go of Eddy, who gave him a withering look. 'So long as you're sure,' the man questioned, but didn't leave Eddy's side.

'Yes, I'm sure. Now are you Ok Eddy?' Sophie asked.

'Yes, I think so,' he said, shaking his head trying to clear his mind.

'It must be very difficult for you because of your… your illness.'

'My illness! Well…Well at least I'm not mad,' Eddy shouted, attracting even more attention from the café customers.

'You're mentally ill Eddy. I expect the tablets obviously help you feel better,' she said gently.

'No they don't…they keep me living in limbo land…I want to be normal…I don't want to be …locked into my head any more,' he implored. 'They can mend broken legs….why can't they mend broken heads?' he demanded angrily.

'Now come on, calm down,' the man said, grabbing Eddy's arm again.

'Get off me ..get off me,' he said shrugging off the man's hand.

'Leave him,' Sophie instructed. 'I'll be alright with him now, thanks.'

'Are you sure Miss?'

'Yeah don't worry. Eddy and I are friends aren't we Eddy?'

'Yes, friends,' Eddy repeated, relieved to hear her confirmation. 'We are very good friends,' he beamed.

'I'll be just over there if you need me,' the man said. …'and we'll be keeping our eye on the phantom chocolate thrower here…right Bruce,' he said, patting Eddy on the shoulder.

'Get off me,' Eddy shrugged the other's hand off.

'OK Eddy now take a deep breath,' Sophie instructed.

'I don't want to be here…I want to run away and …' Eddy filled up. A tear ran down his cheek.

'At least here you can go out when you want to,' she reasoned, fearful that she might lose her freshly found inside source.

'I suppose,' he accepted.

'Anyway, I would imagine that the hospital needs to keep you and the other patients all together for your own protection...You've seen what those yobs, those protesters are like. They are called the normal ones. But they attacked you didn't they?'

'Yes they did. Why did they attack me? I didn't do anything to them.' Eddy asked innocently.

'Because they don't understand...because they are frightened of their own shadow. They're the ones that need locking up,' Sophie added. 'Now tell me about the Professor and Doctor John.'

'Please don't tell them about this,' he begged. 'They will put me back on one of the wards. I don't want to be locked in them anymore. I am better. Honest I am, honest,' he pleaded.

'Ok, I promise. But you've got to help me find stuff about the Professor and the Doctor,' she told him.

'Why?'

'Because...ummm they might get a special award for their work,' she lied. 'But perhaps not the sort that they would appreciate, if she could scandalise their activities,' she thought.

'An award! They would like that wouldn't they? Ok, I promise,' Eddy agreed.

'Good. Now I need to go and change,' she said standing up.

'I'd better leave too,' Eddy said glimpsing at the man who had held him.

'I'll meet you here tomorrow at the same time and let you know exactly what I need, Sophie smiled, pleased with progress.'

Chapter Thirty-four

As he followed Sophie out of the café. Eddy bumped into Marilyn.

'I saw you through the window. Have you been talking to that woman again?' she demanded, menacingly.

'Y...Yes,' Eddy replied sheepishly.

'I told you to keep away from her. She is a nasty woman,' Marilyn dictated.

'She only wants to be friendly,' Eddy said meekly.

'She will get you into trouble. That sort always wants something,' she repeated her warning.

'Listen. Can you hear that?' Eddy asked listening intensely.

'Don't change the subject.'

'I wasn't. I can hear shouting, can you?' Eddy said fearfully. 'Quick, let's go back home,' he said grabbing her hand.

'You don't need to be afraid. I'll protect you,' Marilyn assured him.

Just then a small group of local yobs rushed towards them, shouting. 'There's some more of them. Let's get 'em.'

'Oh no, not again,' Eddy screamed in panic.

'It's Ok Eddy,' Marilyn reassured, stepping in front of him. 'Ok if you want some, come and get it,' she shouted, running towards the yobs menacingly, with her clenched fists raised.

With lightning speed, belying her rounded frame, she managed to deliver a few blows to one of them, a weedy character, before they all backed off.

Taken aback by her unexpected assault, the mob then scattered, but not before someone threw a glass bottle at her.

The bottle hit Marilyn on the shoulder and immediately smashed. Shards of glass flew off the broken bottle and sliced into Marilyn's neck, severing her carotid artery.

Marilyn put her hand up to her neck and realised that she was bleeding heavily. She screamed as she felt the blood pumping out through her fingers dousing her clothes.

Understandably, she went into hysterics and sank to her knees screaming, watching her life blood spurting on to the pavement.

'Eddy, help me. Help me I'm bleeding,' she screamed.

Eddy stared at her in horror. His protector was badly hurt. He was now undefended, vulnerable.

'I have to do something,' he thought frantically, watching blood gushing out of the gash on Marilyn's neck.

And without further thought, he dropped to his knees, took his handkerchief out of his pocket, forced her hands out of the way and quickly pushed the hankie on to the wound. He put his hands around her neck, to try to keep the handkerchief in place and maintain digital pressure to staunch the blood flow.

The horrified café owner, who had already witnessed Eddy's incident with Sophie earlier, was alerted by all the shouting.

Horrified when she saw the blooded Marilyn on the floor and immediately assumed Eddy had gone berserk again and had attacked her. She made an urgent call to the emergency services.

The call generated the despatch of a nearby Police patrol car to the scene within a few minutes.

By the time the Policeman had arrived a small crowd had gathered around Eddy and his patient, Marilyn.

As he pulled up at the scene, the Policeman's initial assessment was that a murder was actively taking place. A man was kneeling over a woman with his hands around her throat. She was laying on her back in a large pool of blood.

'Christ my first solo job and someone is being murdered,' he muttered.

Constable Barry Noland recognised the man as Eddy. As he got out of the car, he withdrew his pistol out of its holster and shouted a warning. 'Armed police, put your hands on your head...and move away from the lady.'

'I can't 'rasped Eddy, his wild eyes gazing at the blood still cascading over his fingers, soaking Marilyn's track suit top.

Desperately the Policeman tried to remember his training. *'In case of hidden firearms, stay crouched behind the open patrol car door.'*

The rookie Policeman, repeated the order. 'Armed police. Eddy put your hands on your head...and move away from the lady.'

The outstretched pistol waivered as he waited for Eddy to comply.

'I can't...I can't, she's going to die,' Eddy shouted, ignoring the command.

'If you don't stand back, I WILL shoot', the PC heard himself say nervously.

Eddy still didn't move.

The Policeman assumed that Eddy's failure to comply meant that he was intending to continue his murderous assault on the woman. Perhaps it was Eddy who stabbed his fellow patient and not Marilyn after all.

The rookie Constable was now in an awful dilemma. Here was the hardest decision of his new Police career. He had been taught the technique of shooting a suspect but was not prepared for the gravity of taking the shot.

The policeman's head was all over the place. Should he shoot or not?

'The sergeant would know what to do,' he thought.

'As he was the first Policeman on scene and with no marksman to take out the target, surely he had to shoot,' he argued with himself.

He was too focussed on the drama to recognise his own fear, heart hammering, dry mouth, adrenaline coursing through him....he had to do it...had to do it.... kill if necessary, fleetingly he remembered his training 'aim for the largest mass'.

He made a judgement that Eddy obviously couldn't have a weapon and therefore he moved away from the car.

Cautiously though, he started moving towards the 'aggressor' and victim to ensure that he could hit his target without causing any collateral casualties.

'Step away or I WILL shoot,' he repeated, targeting Eddy's chest.

Arms outstretched and locked; muscles taunt; his gun like a compass needle attracted to a magnet, as he circumnavigated them.

Then he recognised that the victim underneath him was Eddy's friend Marilyn.

'I'm trying to stop the bleeding,' Eddy explained. 'She was attacked. She's been cut by a broken bottle that someone threw. I'm trying to stop the bleeding,' Eddy repeated, much to the officer's relief.

'Thank god I didn't shoot,' he thought.

Just then an ambulance arrived and pulled up in a cloud of tyre smoke. As the crew got out they quickly assessed the situation and seeing the Policeman with his gun drawn, held back.

'Is it Ok to go to the casualty, constable?' the driver asked.

'Yes. He tells me he is conducting first aid,' the young Policeman said, holstering his pistol.

'I have to keep the pressure on her neck. It's called digital pressure,' Eddy recited.

'Yes. That's correct,' the Ambulance driver confirmed, kneeling next to him. 'Can I help you? Take over from you perhaps?' the paramedic asked, cautiously.

'No, I think...I think it's stopping, but you can set up a saline drip for her shock,' Eddy suggested. 'She has lost a lot of blood.'

'Oh so you know something about dealing with this type of injury do you?' the ambulance man said, impressed by Eddy's knowledge.

'I suppose so, I can't remember where I learnt it though,' Eddy confessed. 'I only know that it's what I was taught.'

'Taught! Who taught you?' the paramedic quizzed, as he busied himself with the saline drip.

'I…I'm not sure. But I know that I need to keep the pressure on her neck…he told me. When I try to remember who, my head feels funny.'

'Was it someone in the crowd?' the ambulance man said trying to make light conversation.

'No, it's the voice, the voice in my head,' Eddy told the sceptical paramedic.

'Eddy is a resident of the sheltered housing,' the Policeman explained quickly to the paramedic.

'Oh, I see,' the ambulance man said knowingly, realising that Eddy was a psychiatric patient.

'How did you get here so quickly, ' the Policeman asked. 'I only just arrived myself.'

'Fortunately we were parked up nearby. Apparently the café owner heard some shouting and screaming and saw Eddy with this lady. Assumed he was killing her.'

'No it was a group of yobs, they attacked us,' Eddy explained earnestly. 'Marilyn hit one of them so they ran away but someone threw a bottle at her and it cut her neck.'

'So Eddy, you're not the villain after all then?' the Policeman surmised.

'No, I was looking after my good friend Marilyn that's all,' Eddy added hastily.

'Did you see her assailant?' the Policeman asked.

'No I was too scared. I didn't want to look. I only heard the shouting and then I heard Marilyn scream that she was bleeding and I saw her lying on the ground,' Eddy added all in a rush. 'So I started first aid with my handkerchief. I stuffed it against the wound and applied pressure to stop the bleeding.'

'Well hopefully you acted in time. Her blood pressure is stable,' the ambulance man advised them. 'Although, she's passed out.'

'Poor Marilyn. Is she going to be OK?' Eddy asked, concerned for his friend.

'Yes, I think so. We'll just finish putting the drip in and get your patient to hospital Eddy,' the ambulance man explained, 'If that's Ok?' he said, seeking Eddy's compliance.

'Yes. Thank you,' Eddy confirmed.

'I'm sure the young lady will thank you when she recovers too. Thanks to your fast reaction, you have saved her life,' the much relieved Policeman observed.

'Marilyn is my best friend.'

'Do you want to come in the ambulance with her?' the ambulance driver asked Eddy.

'Oh yes please,' Eddy beamed.

Chapter Thirty-five

John rushed to the Professors office on the fourth floor with the news. He knocked and without waiting for an invitation to enter, stepped in.

The Professor looked up from his work.

'G'day John. What's all the rush?'

'I've just heard that there has been an incident in town,' John informed him. 'One of our patients has been injured.'

'Oh dear. Do we know who?' the Senior academic asked.

'Yes, it's Eddy's bodyguard, Marilyn.'

'Is she badly hurt?'

'I don't know. But she has gone to hospital in an ambulance.'

'Do you know what her injuries are?' the Professor quizzed.

'Neck injury, apparently,' John informed him.

'Oh dear, any idea what happened?

'Apparently, someone threw a bottle which smashed and cut her badly.'

'Do we know who injured her? Not one of our clients was it?' the Professor probed.

'No, but the Police are investigating. I wonder if it's something to do with one of the Protester groups,' John suggested.

'Yes you could be right. In the meantime, I'll ring the hospital and get an update on her condition,' the Professor said, reaching for his phone.

'I was thinking of going to the hospital later anyway' John volunteered.

'Oh, that's a good idea. Save me having to call them. And you'll be able to assess the situation first hand. Good man.'

'No probs.'

'You know, we can never win with these protesters,' the Professor said, 'We're in a 'catch twenty two' situation.'

'What do you mean?'

'As you know, society demands that we do something about people with mental health issues. In the past we locked them away, out of sight. That wasn't right, so we are now deinstitutionalising them. That's not right either because the local population are not prepared to accept them into their communities,' the Professor continued.

'Yes I soon discovered people's polarised views when I started my psychiatry training. Some want us to become patient helpers and on the other hand, part of society wants us to be their jailers,' John observed.

'As you've discovered people with mental health issues exhibit different behaviour patterns which upset parts of the populace,' the Professor stated. 'That unease, I can understand. But as we know, that transition back from institutional life to community living is hard for clients. It takes time.'

'They need help to make the transition from being looked after to living independently,' John agreed. 'When you think of the list of activities needed to regain their independence and self-confidence, it is quite daunting. Obviously, they need practical support to achieve the change.'

'Exactly, the anti-psychiatry crowd don't understand that it takes time. It can't be done in a rush,' the Professor agreed. 'But understandably, the locals don't want people with strange mannerisms wandering around in their communities either.'

'The truth is these people need special care because society will only accept a relatively small deviation from the norm – whatever that norm is,' John observed. 'Their special individuality is not tolerated.'

'Exactly! Unless of course you have money and a smart lawyer then you can get away with being – different. Then you're called eccentric.' The Professor expanded. 'However if you're poor and unwanted, it's a different story. Society demands that you're banged up, away out of sight and sedated to the hilt.'

'Society's problems then magically goes away,' John observed, sceptically.

'Yes of course it does,' the Professor said, echoing John's cynicism,. 'We are the custodians of the 'caring' society, remember.'

'What it really means is that the psychiatry world take care of their problem relatives. So society can get on with their lives.' John pointed out. 'For me, it epitomises the breakdown of the family structure.'

'Indeed, in many cases they don't even care what we do to their relatives. No, so long as we get rid of their family problem, thus relieving them of their responsibilities,' the Professor suggested, vehemently.

'Anyway, where is the anti-psychiatry movement coming from?' John wondered.

'Sadly, it's usually former psychiatric patients that we have helped, or tried to help.' The Professor explained. 'They've decided they didn't like the methods we used to treat them. The founders of the movement have swayed former patients to think, that whilst in our care, their rights were abused.'

'Biting the hand that feeds them, eh?' John suggested sceptically.

'Anytime you get a protest march about anything, it always attracts the oddballs too. The 'know it all' fanatics who haven't done a useful days work in their life.'

'Something like the 'rent – a – mob' protests of the sixties.'

'Yeah, probably something like that. These are the troublemakers who sow false news stories.'

'These anti mental health protesters are getting more visible...lots of stuff appearing on the television too.'

'Could all be done by the same core group though. They usually link their contacts. Any major problems here that they might exploit?' John queried.

'Major? No not yet. But lots of minor incidents like what happened today. You will always get the militants infiltrating these organisations purely for the hell of it. They're there for their own perverted aims....they deflect debate away from the real issues that should be sorted.'

'Like they did in the states with the anti-abortion lobby.'

'Probably the same mob behind the anti-hunting, anti-vivisection campaign in Britain.' John suggested. 'They were infiltrated by 'green' terrorists ....who decided the debate was getting nowhere so they upped the 'ante' and became headline news with arson attacks, bombs etc.'. So this is the climate we work in….we are just another punch bag for society.' John concluded.

'Well you know the old saying…if you can't take a joke, you shouldn't have joined,' the Professor laughed.

'Thanks.'

'Anyway enough of our moans and groans. Being in our privileged position, it does give us an opportunity to…to, shall we say experiment,' the Professor smiled.

'Experiment? What do you mean?' John quizzed.

'Test the boundaries and hopefully find the holy grail of mental illness.'

'You mean to find a cure for all forms of mental illness? Surely, that's an impossible dream?'

The Cellphone interrupted their debate. The Professor answered quickly. 'Phillips here. Ok, just a minute,' the Professor said putting his hand over the mouthpiece. 'Sorry John, a business call from the Scana-Landis Corp.'

'Scana Landis?' John wondered at the unfamiliar name.

'The Pharmaceutical company,' the Professor explained.

The psychiatrist took the hint. 'Ok, I'll go and find out how Eddy and Marilyn are,' he said, leaving.

'I wonder why the Pharmaceutical company are ringing through on his Cellphone. What confidential information doesn't he want me to hear? What's he up to?,' John pondered.

Chapter Thirty-six

After treatment for her neck wound, and against medical advice, Marilyn discharged herself from the hospital. Together with Eddy they went to catch a bus back to the sheltered housing complex.

'Are you sure that you are well enough,' Eddy asked concerned. 'You lost a lot of blood.'

'Yes, I'll be alright, just a bit sore and whoosy, but I'm tough,' she reassured him. 'Wait til I see those yobs again. They'll be sorry.'

'Oh, no more violence, please. It frightens me,' Eddy confessed.

'We can't let the bullies get the better of us,' Marilyn decreed.

They arrived at the bus stop just in time.

'Here's the bus Marilyn,' Eddy said, as the single decker came into view.

The bus stopped, the doors opened and the pair stepped onto the platform.

'We want to go to Waratara Road,' Marilyn demanded.

The driver hesitated, seeing Eddy and Marilyn's bloodstained clothing, unsure about his new passengers.

'Well?' Marilyn questioned. 'What are you waiting for?.

'OK...mmm...that's ten dollars for the pair of you,' he croaked.

'We don't have to pay. You know that,' Marilyn informed him.

'What are you talking about ?' the driver barked. 'What do you mean, you don't have to pay? Of course you do.'

'You know we don't have to pay,' she repeated.

'Look 'sport', you either pay or you get off my bus,' he said firmly.

'Don't take that attitude with me,' Marilyn ranted. 'We don't pay and that's final,' she repeated, turning as if to take a seat.

'Unless you've got a special pass, you either give me money or you get off the bus. Make up your mind,' the driver insisted.

'I've blonde hair,' Marilyn said, stroking her hair.

'What you on about? For all I care you can have purple eyes and pigtails,' the exasperated driver said. 'Money or off.'

'We blonde haired people are superior to you, I read it in a book,' she continued.

'You ain't blonde...you've dyed it...and not very well either,' the driver pointed out. 'You look like a haystack on the turn.'

'Aryans are superior. We are the master race,' she informed him.

'Well I think in your case, something went wrong,' he said cruelly. 'Now off the bus before I call the police.'

'We shall stay here until you get us to our destination,' Marilyn told him firmly. 'Won't we Eddy?'

'If you say so,' Eddy said meekly, feeling uncomfortable at the confrontation. All the time he was wondering what Marilyn was up to, as he had never seen her like this before.

'Oh yeah and where's your actual destination, as if I didn't know.'

'We are special people. We live in special houses,' Marilyn explained.

'With special keepers,' the bus driver added, cruelly.

'They are our servants,' Marilyn said haughtily. 'They look after our every needs.'

'Enough of this nonsense! Get off my bus,' the driver exploded. 'I haven't got all day, and there's people who have paid and want to get home.'

As if on cue an irate passenger shouted from the back of the bus. 'Driver what's the hold up?'

'Oh just a little problem with someone who wants a free ride,' the driver informed him, glaring at Marilyn and Eddy.

'I don't have to pay,' Marilyn shouted, hoping to elicit sympathy from the passenger.

But her appeal failed and instead the passenger shouted, 'Well get off the frigging bus. I want to get home to my family.'

'No I shall stay here until the driver fulfils my needs.'

'I'll fulfil your bleedin' needs with a black eye if you don't move, the irate passenger said standing.

'Ok Sir, I'll handle this. No need to get excited,' the driver said calmly.

'Excited! Excited! Of course I'm bloody excited. I've had a hard day at work and now I just want to get home. And you're taking orders from a delusional woman. Now are you going to throw them off or am I?' the passenger demanded.

'Well at this rate, none of us will be going anywhere until the Police arrive,' the driver added reaching for his radio.

'That's bloody typical isn't it…are you satisfied now you…you bleedin nutter,' the passenger said, walking towards the pair.

'Come on Marilyn, let's get off. I don't think that you're very well.' Eddy said, grabbing her arm. 'She's not very well,' Eddy implored. 'She was attacked and has just come out of the hospital.'

'If she doesn't move, she will be going back there too,' the passenger warned.

'Don't you pick on me,' Marilyn said pulling herself up to her full five foot six. 'I've my secret police everywhere. They will deal with you. You will be sorry,' she threatened. 'I'll go and summon my troops. You will wait here.' she said, finally leading Eddy off the bus.

'Ok. Now they've gone. Let's get the hell out of here, 'the passenger demanded.

'You don't have to ask twice,' the driver said, hitting the button to close the doors and ramming the bus into gear.

As the bus pulled away Marilyn shouted at the departing vehicle.

'I told you to wait. I've got your number….my troops will stop you at the roadblock. You'll be sorry.'

'Come on Marilyn, you're not very well. Perhaps we ought to go back to the hospital?' Eddy said, frightened by his friend's irrational behaviour.

Suddenly, she started staring at the grass verge.

'Oh look Eddy, look at that. The grass is really green, I've never seen grass so green before.....have you?'

Marilyn squealed. The sudden dip in her blood pressure was obviously causing confusion in her drugged brain.

Eddy looked at her sympathetically and put his arm around her shoulders.

'I expect that it was the drugs they gave you at the hospital that has made you go a bit cranky. Losing all that blood must have upset your blood pressure too. Come on Marilyn, we'll walk home instead,' he said, compassionately, holding her hand and leading them down the road.

Just as they started walking, John pulled up in his new car and wound down the passenger window.

'Hello you two,' he said. 'I was just coming to see if you were Ok. Are you on your way home?'

'Yes.'

'Ok, let me give you a lift.'

'Thank you doctor,' the pair chorused.

'I see by your bloody clothes that you've both had a bit of a problem,' he observed sympathetically.'

'Yes, we were attacked by some yobs and Eddy saved my life using first aid, Marilyn revealed sounding lucid.

'Well done Eddy. First aid eh? Where did you learn that?' John asked.

'I don't know. Before I knew it, I was just doing it. Isn't that strange?'

'Well the important thing is that you used it and saved a life,' John pointed out. 'Very well done.'

'Thank you,' Eddy said modestly.

'Come on, get in then. Don't worry about messing the car up, I haven't removed the plastic covering from the seats yet, although I wasn't expecting to have passengers so soon.'

The pair climbed into John's new BMW 3 Series E30 which he had selected for its all-wheel drive.

'We'll soon be back and I'll have a quick look at the hospitals work on your neck Marilyn,' John said.

'Thank you doctor.'

'Then I suggest that you both have an early night,' John said as he turned the car.

'This is a nice car Doctor,' Eddy said, stroking the dashboard.

'Yes, I'm very pleased with it. It's the 325iX model and has a 2 litre, six cylinder petrol engine under the bonnet,' the Doctor informed him.

The group were silent for the rest of the journey as John drove them home.

Eddy was reliving the very frightening and bloody events of the day as Marilyn was planning revenge on her assailant.

Chapter Thirty-seven

It took several weeks of painstaking research by Laura to track down information about Eddy's father's career.

The quarter of a century since the traumatic events meant that information was very sparse. Consequently she wasted a lot of time on many false leads, until at last she finally hit the jackpot.

As Laura entered John's office, her beaming smile signalled her success. It was obvious that she was bursting to tell him the results of her findings.

'Looks like you might have some good news for me then Laura,' he said, as she sat down in front of him.

'Yes I have,' she smiled. 'Eddy's father was indeed a GP in Sydney, as you had speculated. The source of my information is another Doctor. His name is Dominic Strong and at the time he was a junior colleague to Eddy's father, Doctor Justin Jones.

Indeed, Dominic became a friend of the family and knew about Eddy's tragic life too,' Laura explained. Fortunately, his memory was incredibly sharp, so he was able to provide a lot of details.

'Brilliant, good news indeed,' the psychiatrist told her.

'Well, following the accident, Eddy was alone with his injured father for…two whole days and nights…as you know he was only a kid…a ten year old,' Laura confirmed.

'God what a trauma for the kid that must have been…alone with his severely injured father for that length of time. No wonder he has problems,' John concluded.

'Apparently the family had emigrated to OZ several years prior to the accident and were well liked in the ex-pats community,' Laura explained. 'Although the step-mum was viewed as a bit of a strange character, Justin excused her mannerisms by telling everyone that she was just homesick.'

'That couldn't have been easy for them all then.

'No. She obviously didn't settle in like husband and son did.'

'Anyway, the move to OZ confirms what Eddy told me under hypnosis,' John revealed.

'Dominic told me that apparently, they had to leave the UK because of matrimonial baggage from Justin's first marriage.

'What do you mean?

'Although he was married, he had a bit of a reputation of fraternising with the staff at work,' Laura explained.

'So are you saying that he and the step mother worked together at the same practice?' John quizzed.

'Yes. And what is even worse. While Doctor Jones' wife was in the delivery suite having their second child, he was being unfaithful with this woman, who became Eddy's step-mother,' Laura said distastefully.

'A bit of a Don Juan then?'

'I'd call him something less flattering,' Laura said angrily. He was obviously a lecher. How could anyone do that while his wife was giving birth to his child?' she added indignantly.

'Despicable character, I agree,' John concurred.

'So, understandably when Eddy's Mum found out about the affair, she was devastated,' Laura continued.

'It must have been awful for her.'

'On top of that, unfortunately, Eddy's mother suffered from post-natal depression too. Then shortly after, the marriage broke down and Eddy's parents separated and the Doctor moved in with his mistress.

'Bad start for the kids,' John said, sympathetically.

Sadly Eddy's Mum just couldn't cope alone with having a toddler and a baby,' Laura revealed.

'That's so sad. Just at a point in her life when she should be enjoying the pleasures of motherhood, her world falls apart.' John said sympathetically. Sadly, I see a lot of patients with similar situations in my consulting rooms.'

'So, as a result of the symptoms of her depression, Doctor Justin was granted custody of Eddy, his toddler son.'

'Split the family then?'

'Yes and then after a few years, the bastard, pardon my language, further twisted the knife in his former wife's guts by emigrating here to OZ with his mistress, now wife, thus removing all contact between mother and Eddy,' Laura relayed harshly.

'So Eddy's birth Mother was left back in England with a young baby?' John observed. 'How tragic.'

'Yeah. From what I could gather. Step mother and Eddy didn't get on too well either, so little Eddy became his father's constant companion. Doctor Justin would even take him out on house calls to his patients' Laura continued. 'You get the picture? Apparently the two were inseparable.'

'Yes, I can see how devastating it would have been for Eddy,' John agreed.

'Anyway, moving on to the crash; when the rescuers found the pair at the crash site, the father was trapped in the wreckage, but had received first aid...it turned out the little boy had done it all...under his father's directions...' Laura relayed.

'Impressive. There's not many kids that could have done that. Did the father survive?'

'No. Sadly his father died, apparently just minutes after they got him to hospital.

But, they reckon that Eddy blamed himself for not doing enough to save his father and hence his guilt trip.'

'Christ! But he was only a kid,' John observed. 'His guilt would be made even worse because of this incredible father and son bond that they appear to have had. It would have been an unimaginable psychological stress for him.'

'Even for an adult it would have been awful, let alone for a scared child,' Laura said, filling up. And you're right, it sounds like that he burdened himself with that guilt. Nothing any of Justin's colleagues could say would dissuade him from this thought,' Laura continued.

'He was obviously traumatised and deeply in shock then, poor kid. Did your informant say what they did for him?'

'Well, they medicated him with anti-depressants. But nothing seemed to work. He got progressively more and more depressed and withdrawn,' Laura revealed.

'Well I suppose you can't blame them, in those days Post Traumatic Stress Disorder was not well understood,' John explained.

'So the worse he got ...the more medication he had. My source said it was sad to see. Eventually, he became totally dependent on his drugs to even get out of bed,' Laura enlarged.

'Poor kid. But didn't I read somewhere that Eddy's step mother was a nurse,' John observed.

'Yes, she was.'

'Well, so what happened to her after the accident? Surely she was around to look after Eddy? John probed.

'Apparently, she couldn't cope with the loss of her husband and the challenge of Eddy's psychiatric problems. It all became too much and she too became depressed.'

'So do we know what happened to her?' John queried.

'My source wasn't sure. She disappeared from the scene, leaving Eddy with Dominic's family.'

'For how long?'

'She never came back.'

'Did they search for her?'

'Yes but never found her, It was rumoured that she might have committed suicide or even gone back to England. But because of her unfriendly nature, nobody appeared to have tried to track her down,' Laura said quietly. 'Obviously it meant that Eddy was all alone with a strange family.'

'Did Dominic adopt him?'

'No, he stayed with them for a short time but after a while they couldn't cope with his unpredictable behaviour and he went into care.'

'Poor kid. Hence the start of the foster homes and institutions,' John acknowledged. 'That's heartbreaking. The whole family destroyed by that terrible accident.'

'Yes, so sad,' Laura said, a lump in her throat.

'Anyway you have uncovered some excellent background information. Thank you. Now all we need to do is to find the actual crash site for a pilgrimage,' John said.

'Yes, I'm still on that. But I thought you'd like to hear about Eddy's background first,' Laura revealed, wiping away a tear.

'Well done, that's brilliant research. I can use that to steer my questions during my next session with Eddy. Thank you.' John said, going to her and giving her a reassuring hug. 'Let's hope we can help him get his life back on track,' John said quietly.

'I hope so too,' Laura said thickly. 'I hope so.'

Chapter Thirty-eight

Despite the Professor's concerns about John's proposed hypnotherapy treatment and any possible undesirable consequences, John was still keen to go ahead and find the trigger that would remove the road block to Eddy's recall.

Although, having been warned by the great man, he was mindful that he was 'skating on thin ice' whilst exorcising Eddy's memories, and could, conceivably cause some additional issues.

So with the information from the file and the feedback that Laura had unearthed at his fingertips John arranged for another hypnotherapy session with Eddy.

Eddy arrived punctually at John's office.

'Good morning Eddy. Are you and Marilyn Ok after that terrible incident the other day?' the psychiatrist asked.

'Marilyn had a stiff neck and I am scared someone might attack us again,' he said fearfully.

'I'm sure that it was just a one off incident Eddy. The police have increased the number of patrols around here at the Professor's insistence. So hopefully that will keep the yobs at bay.'

'Oh, that's good. It was very scary,' Eddy admitted. 'Especially after I was knocked down as well.'

'I'm sure that it was. But you did a good job with that first aid,' John reassured him. 'You most certainly saved Marilyn's life.'

'Thank you,' Eddy said, sitting down on the couch. 'Did you know that she went a bit…a bit funny just before you picked us up.'

'No. What happened?'

'Well we were catching a bus and she pretended that we didn't have to pay and told the bus driver she was an Aryan, whatever that is. And then she was ranting about the colour of the grass.'

'Probably an episode brought on by the shock,' John suggested.

'You don't think it's anything to do with the pills the Professor is giving us do you?' Eddy asked. 'Because I had a funny turn the other day too.'

'Well, I suppose it might be. In any case it needs to be reported so that the drug side effects can be identified.'

'The Professor wasn't interested when I told him about my funny turn though,' Eddy revealed.

'Are you sure Eddy? Perhaps he didn't understand what you were saying?'

'No he said it was just one of those things.'

'Mmm that's suspicious,' John thought. Although he didn't know the prescribed medication that Eddy was taking; surely it was vital to capture all side effects?

'Well the Professor knows what he's doing,' John pointed out, although unsure whether there wasn't a bit of skulduggery going on.

'I thought Marilyn's problem might have been the loss of blood and low blood pressure that caused it,' Eddy explained.

John was surprised at Eddy's lucid explanation. 'He obviously has a thinking brain in there somewhere,' John thought. 'Hopefully soon, we'll be able to release it from the damage of years of misdiagnosis.'

'Right, if you're ready to start, would you like to sit on the couch?'

'Ok,' Eddy said, positioning himself.

'So if you're comfortable, is it Ok to start?' John asked.

'Yes, thanks. Do you think you will find the answers today?' Eddy queried.

'No. But I think this will be another step forward in uncovering things in your past. Let's put the EEG cap on then.'

'Ok.'

After putting the multi-wired cap on Eddy's head, John quickly put him into a trance.

Satisfied that he was deeply under, the hypnotherapist directed his questions straight to what he considered was Eddy's hidden secret and the cause for his initial illness.

'Remember you are Eddy's observer,' John reminded his unconscious patient, 'Does Eddy remember a car crash?'

'No,' Eddy tensed. The EEG reflected his discomfort.

'He was alone with his Daddy for several days in a crashed car,' John reminded Eddy.

'No, it's not to be talked about.' Eddy squirmed.

'Why Eddy? If we talk about it. Eddy's headaches will get better and it won't hurt so much.'

Eddy started to cry; tears rolled down his cheeks.

'Take your time Eddy,' the hypnotherapist encouraged gently. 'Nothing will hurt you. You are safe here.'

'They couldn't save his Dad. Eddy kept him alive until help came. Eddy was his Dad's only hope, he'd told him that. And he failed his father,' he sobbed.

'No he didn't fail him. He was a ten year old child. He was in the middle of nowhere. He did well to keep his Dad alive for so long after the crash.' John reasoned. 'He can't put that pressure on himself.'

'No, I failed him,' Eddy repeated sadly. Now no longer the observer. 'Otherwise he would still be alive.'

'Just relax. Tell me what actually happened. Let your mind drift back all those years. There is nothing there that will hurt you. Just relax Eddy, relax,' John encouraged softly. 'Remember you are the observer. Eddy's observer. Tell me what he experienced.'

Eddy was transported back to the fateful incident.

It was like a dam bursting, as minute details about the incident spilled out as Eddy's observer relayed the story.

'He and his Daddy were going fishing on Lake Jindabyne in the... he thinks it was called the Kosciuszho National Park. He couldn't pronounce it, so instead they called it the Kozy park. They laughed about that,' he smiled in his trance.

'Ah ha, at last a location to work with,' John thought, scribbling it down on his notepad. 'Must let Laura know.'

'They both liked fishing and hoped to get some Salmon or Trout for their tea. It was a long drive from Sydney. He thinks it took them over five hours.'

'I expect that Eddy was excited at the thought of the adventure?' John suggested.

'Yes, he was. Until they got lost looking for their campsite. They were driving down a narrow track. It was great fun because there were ramps on the track and the car kept leaping into the air. Eddy enjoyed the sensation so much that he urged his Dad to go faster and make the car do bigger leaps. They were having great fun until they landed after one big leap and in front of them in the track was a big emu.'

'Oh heavens,' John muttered under his breath.

Eddy tensed up on the couch. 'He shouted. Look out Dad, there's an emu.

But it was too late. Their car slammed into a huge emu. The collision sent the bird over the top of the bonnet and smashed through the windscreen knocking his Daddy out.'

Eddy put his arms up to ward off the imaginary emu.

'The car was going very fast and it went out of control and slammed into a big tree.'

Eddy's brain waves peaked as he unconsciously tensed his hands, whilst reliving the collision.

'He thinks he was knocked out, for the next thing he remembers seeing was the dead Emu lying on top of his Dad.

He shouted Dad; Dad are you alright?...Dad.....but his Daddy didn't answer.'

Eddy became animated in his trance.

'He had difficulty opening his passenger door, it was jammed. But after a struggle, he eventually kicked it open.'

On the couch, Eddy's leg kicked out as if to replicate his actions at the crash site.

He went around to his Daddy's side of the car and yanked open the driver's door. As he did, the huge Emu slithered off Daddy, just missing him. It was horrible, it's guts spilled out on to the floor and the smell was awful. He was nearly sick.

Then he saw that his Daddy was bleeding. He shouted, Dad, you're bleeding….Dad. Don't worry, I'll get help, he said.'

Eddy's hands reflected his hopelessness.

'He ran back up to the road shouting. 'Help, help… please someone help me…help. My Dad's been hurt really bad…Help'. He looked around but there was no houses, no cars on the road or anyone around.

Chapter Thirty-nine

'Nobody came to their help. Eddy was frantic. He was alone with his badly injured Dad. Nobody came along the road, so after a while he ran back to his Daddy in the car.

He remembers crunching over the broken windscreen glass as he got back to his Dad's side. His Daddy was still unconscious.

'Dad, please speak to me, Dad, he said shaking his Daddy's arm. Thankfully, his Daddy stirred. Oh thank goodness you're still alive, he shouted.'

'Oh my head,' his Dad groaned. 'What...what happened...I remember, the Emu...is it Ok, did I miss it?'

'No Dad,' he said. 'The Emu is dead. We crashed very fast into a tree. Dad, you're hurt. You're bleeding really bad from your neck...what can I do, what can I... do?' he was panicking.'

'That must have been terrible. A young kid pitched into an awful situation alone. He was only ten for heaven's sake.' John thought, emotionally absorbed in the phantom child's story.

'His Dad said, Eddy, apart from my head, I can't feel anything. I am all kind of numb at the moment. Where am I bleeding from?' his Dad asked.

'Dad, it's pumping out of your neck…it's running down your shirt. He told him.'

'Ok son, don't worry. But I need you to help …will you do that…? His Dad asked quietly.'

'Yes Dad of course I will. But you won't die will you?' He pleaded. He was very scared.'

'Yes I bet he was,' John acknowledged, under his breath.

'No son, it's Ok,' his Daddy reassured him. 'I won't die. But you'll have to be quick to help me. Do you understand?'

'Yes.'

'In the boot of the car is my medical bag,' he told him. 'Will you get it for me?'

'Yes, Ok'

And he quickly ran to the back of the car and tried to open the boot. 'but he couldn't. I can't Dad,' he shouted. ….it's stuck…it's stuck Dad.' He really tried very hard to open it, using all his strength.'

Again Eddy's hands reflected his recalled efforts.

'I expect you did,' John thought, visualising the young Eddy's struggles.

'Don't worry son. Try the keys. Use the keys to open it. His Daddy said, he was so calm.'

'Where are they ?'

'Here in the ignition, he informed him. But please hurry. If we don't stop the bleeding I shall….'

'No Dad please don't die.' He cried as he ran back to his Daddy and grabbed the keys.

'No, I won't die, but I might pass out.'

'Ok I'm hurrying. He put the keys in the boot lock. Yes, it's opening. He told his Daddy. He was so relieved.'

'Good boy.'

'I've got the bag Dad.' He told his Daddy.
'Good boy…bring it back here.'
'He hurried back to the open driver's door.'
'Now I want you to open the bag and take out a big dressing…remember the sort we practiced first aid on Molly your cat, when we pretended she'd been run over,' his Daddy said.
'He took out the dressing and ripped the bag open. 'I've got it, He told him.'
'Right now, I want you to push it tightly into the place on my neck, where the blood is coming from,' he told Eddy…'Do you think you can do that?'
'Yes,' Eddy said. He was very nervous.'
'Now if I pass out when you do this,' he told him, 'don't worry, you must keep the pressure on until the blood stops. It's called digital pressure ….is that Ok?'
'Yes,' Eddy said and stuffed the dressing into his Daddy's neck wound.
'Ohhh Jeez…that…hurts….' His Dad said and passed out.'
All the while Eddy's hands were twitching as he described his actions.
'Eddy was so scared. He thought he'd killed his Daddy. Dad, Dad, he yelled please don't go to sleep. Dad, please wake up. Dad,' he cried. 'Don't leave me.'
Within a few minutes, his Dad opened his eyes again.' Oh where am I?…his Dad asked.'
'Dad you woke up,' he was so pleased.
'Is it stopping son?' his Dad asked.
'It wasn't. Eddy said I don't think so Dad…oh god, I'm sorry…Dad.'
'You must try harder,' his Dad said. 'Push really hard. Like when you and I play push over.'

'But I don't want to hurt you anymore,' Eddy told him.

'No it's alright...you must push really hard to stop the bleeding,' he encouraged him. 'remember It's called digital pressure.'

'Ok...I'll try,' and Eddy used all his strength to jam the dressing into his Dad's wound

'Ohhh! Keep pushing son. It's the only way to help me.'

'Dad. I'm scared.

'No, it's Ok. You're doing really well,' his Daddy encouraged.

And it finally stopped the bleeding.

Dad It's stopped,' He was so pleased.

'Now I know how he was able to treat Marilyn's injury so successfully.' John thought. 'Well I'll be blowed.'

Eddy continued to relay his story.

'His Dad said well done, I knew you could do it. Now listen. Now I need you to tell me about my other injuries. Do you understand?'

'Yes Dad.'

'You must be brave...I don't know how long it will be before we will be rescued.'

'Ok.'

'As well as not being able to move my arms, I can't feel my legs either.'

'Your legs are trapped. The front of the car has been pushed back and the steering wheel is resting on your chest. Oh Daddy what can I do?'

'I want you to put your other hand on my leg where you can see it...gently....but keep the pressure on my neck.'

'Ok, it's there,' he said.

'No I can't feel it...push down a bit harder,' he told him.

'Ok.

'No still can't feel anything, try the other leg,' his Dad directed.

'My hand is on your other leg.'

'No still can't feel that...Ok...It looks like I've broken my neck.'

'Oh Dad!'

'Now I want you to help me. I need you to put a needle in my arm to put in a drip.'

'No I don't want to hurt you,' he cried.

'But this will help me get better...it will help with the shock. Do you think you can do that ?'

'Ok, he said, but he really didn't want to do it.'

Even in his trance Eddy shook his head as if to emphasise his reluctance.

"You're doing absolutely fine,' his Dad encouraged. 'Now has the bleeding from my neck stopped?...No don't take the dressing off,' he told him, feeling the pressure lift from his neck injury.

'Yes it looks like.' Eddy told him.

'Ok now you need to bandage that on and then we can start on the drip...is that Ok?'

'He was so frightened.'

'But his Dad kept reassuring him. Yes I know son but I need you to be a brave soldier for me now. Just like I looked after you, now it's your turn to look after me.'

'But I can't..'

'Yes you can....if you want to be a doctor someday... now's the time to start with your first patient.

'Ah ha,' John thought. 'So that's where his pretending to be a doctor or Ambulance man has come from. A frustrated career plan cut short. What a pity.'

Eddy continued with the story. 'So Eddy set up a line for a saline drip for dealing with his Dad's shock with the bag hanging off the sun visor.

'But it was the flies. He had to deal with the flies. They are a real nuisance, a nuisance,' he said, swotting invisible insects away. 'The flies are being attracted to the dead Emu. They are all over it.'

'It was then that he smelt it?'

'Smelt what Eddy? The Emu?' John asked.

'No. He can smell smoke. The forest is on fire!' Eddy said and started thrashing around again. 'His Dad is trapped in the car and the forest was on fire. '

The EEG monitor trace was going haywire again and conscious of the Professor's warning, John chose to bring Eddy out of the trance. Hoping that he hadn't already probed too deeply. Eddy's reactions were showing dangerous signs of emotional trauma. The exercise was causing Eddy significant issues as he was sweating profusely too.

'Ok Eddy. Just relax. Come back to me slowly. There is no more to observe. Come away from the car. Relax, you are not in danger. You are feeling better now,' he coaxed. 'Some of the poison that hurt your mind is disappearing. It is time to open your eyes and come back in the room. Gently, slowly,' the psychiatrist intoned.

Eddy came to, his face bathed in sweat.

'You're doing really well,' the psychiatrist encouraged giving him a sterile flannel to wipe his face. '

'I feel exhausted.' Eddy said mopping his brow.' What happened?'

'You're doing really well. We're getting there. Don't worry, we'll get rid of your demons soon,' John said optimistically.

Chapter Forty

Eddy went to meet Sophie outside the café at the agreed time, only to find that she was already inside and seated.

Although he didn't recall what had actually happened, Eddy was still rather 'shaky' from the efforts of the intense hypnotherapy session with John.

Feeling flustered, he hesitantly entered the cafe, expecting to be told by the café owner to leave.

But fortunately the owner was busy, so avoiding any possible eye contact, Eddy headed for Sophie's table, staring at the floor.

'G'day Eddy, how are you today?' she smiled, ingratiating herself to him. 'Take a seat.'

'I'm Ok,' he lied, whilst actually feeling emotionally drained after the events of the previous days.

'Do you want a drink?'

'Umm, I'm not sure,' he said, hesitantly, recalling the previous hot chocolate incident.

'Well, so long as you're not going to throw this one over me, I'll buy you a drink,' she teased.

'In that case, could I have a glass of water?'

'Yes that's probably a good choice. Less likely to end in tears.' Sophie agreed and called the waitress over.

'A cup of black coffee and a small glass of water,' she ordered. The waitress duly departed.

'Right Eddy, I want you to tell me as much as you can about the goings on in the Imagine Institute.

'The Institute! Why do you need to know?' Eddy asked nervously.

'Remember I was talking about the possible awards for the Professor and your Doctor?'

'Oh yes.'

'Well in order for them to qualify I have to make sure that they are treating you correctly,' she lied. 'Some of these institutes have a bad reputation for mistreating their patients.'

'Oh, Ok. Well I think they are very good there,' he replied. 'What do you want me to say?'

'I'll ask some questions and if you don't know the answer, don't worry. You will just have to go and find out for me. Is that understood?' she checked, getting a small tape recorder out of her pocket.

'Yes,' Eddy said, uneasily. 'What's that?' he asked suspiciously, staring at the recorder.

'It's only a tape recorder. Nothing to worry about,' she assured him. 'It helps me remember what you said, when I write up my notes, that's all.'

At this stage, the waitress brought their drinks and Sophie paid, putting the bill in her purse. After the waitress had gone, Sophie started her interrogation.

'Right, let's start then. Some of the information you have already told me, but I just want to get it recorded in your voice. Is that OK?

'Yes.'

'Eddy, who is on the drug trial?' Sophie asked.

'Drug trial?' Eddy repeated, trying to think what she meant. 'Oh the drug trial! Why everyone in our special houses are,' he revealed. 'I don't know who else is on it.'

'Good. How many is that?' she continued.

Eddy scratched his head. 'Well…ummm…Let me think,' he said, gazing at the ceiling. Umm… it was twelve, I think, until some disappeared.'

'Disappeared! How many have disappeared?' she demanded, feeling excited that she was at last going to be able to record first-hand information of the possible link with the Professor's treatments.

'Umm…three people,' Eddy revealed.

'What are their names?'

'Umm…let me think now. There was Digger…umm Peter and umm…what was his name? Mathew, that's right Mathew.'

'Well done. Now what were their last names?'

'Last names? I don't know. None of us around here know anybody's last name.'

'Ok, no problem. But can you find out for me?'

'I don't know how to do that,' he said.

'Well surely, there's an office in the Institute?. They will have records,' she said brusquely. 'You could try there.'

'Oh, Ok,' Eddy said, awkwardly; wondering how he would get in the office, as it was out of bounds to all patients. But he was frightened to tell her so.

'What is the drug that you are taking?' she continued.

'I don't know. We are just handed the pill,' he revealed.

'Then you will have to find a way of getting it for me,' she said, forcefully.

'Ok, but how?'

'I don't know. There must be bottles around when they are handing them out. You will just have to keep your eyes open,' she said forcefully.

'Oh, Ok.'

'Do you know if the Professor and the Doctor are working together on the trial?'

'No, I don't know. But the Doctor hasn't been here long.'

'Well that's something else to add to your list then,' she instructed. 'There's a lot more questions that I have but I doubt that you would be able to answer them.'

'Thank you,' he said relieved.

'Perhaps I need to have words with your doctor friend to provide that additional information.'

'Yes, that would be a good idea,' he agreed, pleased to duck out of the interrogation.'

'Let me have those answers as soon as possible. Say by five days' time and we'll meet in the park, Ok?' Sophie suggested.

'Ok,' Eddy said meekly, but having already forgotten her requirements he had to ask again.

'Sorry, but what did I have to find out?' he asked uncomfortably, expecting to be told off.

'Oh, don't worry. I'll write it down for you,' she said exasperated. 'Can you read?'

'Yes of course,' he replied defensively, feeling hurt that she doubted his literary capabilities.

She called it out as she wrote each one down. 'Surnames of the missing; Name of the drug; Is the new doctor working on the trial?' Got it now?' she said, handing him the neatly written note.

'Yes thank you,' he smiled.

She patted his hand patronisingly, they finished their drinks and left.

Chapter Forty-one

Several days after his meeting with Sophie and wondering how he was going to provide her with the information that she wanted, Eddy attended John's consulting room for his next hypnotherapy session.

'G'day Doctor, nice to see you,' Eddy gushed, thinking the session gave him the excuse to be in the building. This would be his chance to hopefully get in to the records office, to get the information that the woman, he knew as Sheila, wanted.

'Nice to see you too Eddy. How does it feel to be a hero?'

'What do you mean, hero?' Eddy puzzled.

'Remember you saved Marilyn's life the other day with a bit of fast first aid,' John reminded him. 'Well that was heroic, keeping your head and saving her life.'

'I've never been called a hero before. A hero!; he repeated the word and smiled. 'I just somehow knew what to do,' Eddy said, warming to the hero label.

'You knew exactly what to do because you'd done it before,' John revealed.

'Done it before? Had I? I...I...don't really know. I can't remember doing it before,' Eddy puzzled.

'That's interesting,' John thought. 'Although he recalled the very fine details of the incident under hypnosis, Eddy had no memory recall now. Fascinating. His brain is still trying to protect him,' he concluded.

'Well the Police and Ambulance people were very impressed. I gather that you even told the paramedics to put in a saline drip.'

'Yes, I did, didn't I?'

'You must have been trained sometime,' the Psychiatrist said, hoping to trigger some form of recall of Eddy's revelations from the previous hypnotherapy session.

'No. Can't remember,' Eddy said, shaking his head.

'Anyway, how were you after our last session,' the psychiatrist asked. 'You looked exhausted.'

'I was quite shaky. But I didn't have any nightmares this time.'

'Oh that's really good.'

'But I keep smelling smoke.'

'Smoke! That's interesting,' The psychiatrist thought. 'As I recall you did mention that towards the end of the previous session.'

'Did I?' Eddy said surprised.

'Yes you did,' John confirmed.

'That's a good sign of the effectiveness of the sessions,' he thought, recalling the contents of the newspaper article, which reported that Eddy and his father had been rescued from an advancing forest fire.

'Well let's see how far we can get today. If you'd like to take your place on the couch as usual,' the psychiatrist invited.

Eddy lay down, now feeling comfortable with the process. Within a few minutes he was attached to the EEG monitor and in a trance.

'Ok Eddy, I am going to take you back, back through the years, back to the inside of the crashed car with your Dad still trapped inside. Remember, he has just told you that you must look after him. Take your time and, as the observer tell me what happened next to Eddy.'

Eddy twisted and turned. The skull cap relaying the internal battle that Eddy was having recalling the hidden childhood horror.

'Nice and slowly Eddy,' the psychiatrist encouraged softly. 'That's it, I can see you are winning. Eddy has connected his Dad to the drip, what happened next?'

'He could smell smoke,' observer Eddy revealed.

'Was the car on fire?'

'No. It…it…the smoke was drifting through the trees and getting thicker. Suddenly he heard noises in the forest, getting louder and louder coming towards them.'

'Noises! What sort of noises was it?'

'Running noises.

Was it somebody coming to their assistance?'

'That's what Eddy thought at first. We are going to be saved.'

'And was it?'

'No. It was animals….'

'What sort of animals?'

'Flocks of emu. Stampeding away from the fire.'

'I expect Eddy was scared to see them?'

'Yes he was. Some of the emus emerged through the forest very close to their car.'

'What did he do?'

'After a while, the stampede stopped. He told himself that he needed to get help. By then he could see through a gap in the trees, planes and helicopters flying overhead.

So he thought he needed to build a big S.O.S on the ground so search planes could see that they needed help.'

'That was good thinking. How did he make the SOS sign,' John probed.

'Stones. He used a lot of big stones laid on the ground to form the letters.'

'Eddy wondered, If they were fighting the forest fire, would they have time to come and search for them anyway?'

'The waiting must have been awful for him. What about the heat?' John asked.'

'It was already so hot in the car. He kept fanning his Dad to cool him down.'

Eddy's hands demonstrated a fanning action.

'The smoke. The smoke was getting thicker and he could hear the crackling of the fire getting louder.'

Eddy coughed as if he was still immersed in the smoke.

'How long were they there before they were rescued?'

'They were in the wreckage for two days without being discovered and all the time the fire was getting closer and closer and the smoke was getting thicker and thicker.'

'I expect that he was scared.'

'Yes. he was. He was frightened that the fire would reach them before anyone would find them and they'd die,' Eddy said quietly.

'What about his father, was he conscious?'

'He kept drifting in and out of consciousness and making funny noises in his sleep.'

'Understandable with the injuries that he had suffered. What did Eddy do to help him?

'He changed the empty saline bottle,' Eddy gesticulated with his hands.

'Well done.'

'He also kept flicking the flies off. It was very difficult even though he had moved the dead Emu further away. The flies were attracted to the blood on his clothes.'

'Did Eddy have anything to eat or drink?'

'Yes, they had brought some food and lots of water for their camping plans.'

'How far away was the forest fire now?'

'It's getting closer and closer. When it got dark he could see the sky was orange from the flames and there were millions of sparks flying up in the air.'

'So can he remember the moment when the rescue came?'

'Yes. He was sitting holding his Dad's hand and he could hear a vehicle coming. He got excited and shouted, Dad, Dad we're saved. Someone is coming. He was so happy. He ran out onto the track. It was a big fire engine. It stopped near their car.'

Chapter Forty-two

'The firemen got out and looked at Eddy in amazement. They shouted. 'What the hell are you doing here? Don't you know the forest is on fire?'

'Eddy said, 'can you help us please. We had an accident and my Daddy is badly hurt. He's trapped in the car.'

'So the SOS spotted by the air crew was genuine,' the fireman said. 'Thank goodness we didn't ignore it. In all honesty we weren't expecting to find anyone,' the leading fireman revealed.

Overcoming their surprise, the firemen quickly examined the wreck and could see that his Daddy was in a bad way.'

'I bet that Eddy was happy that at last something was going to happen,' John suggested. And that his father was going to receive proper medical assistance at last?'

'Yes he was. As some of the fire crew got equipment out to release his Dad from the wreckage, the Leader got on their radio and called for a helicopter to evacuate them.

'So how long did they wait for the helicopter to arrive?'

'He doesn't know, but it seemed like forever. While they were waiting the firemen cut his Daddy out of the wrecked car. When they had to move Daddy from the wreck. He screamed a lot. It was horrible.'

'I expect Eddy was even more frightened hearing his father's screams?'

'Yes, he was. He put his hands over his ears and ran and hid behind the fire engine.

In his trance Eddy emulated his description and put his hands over his ears.

'When the helicopter arrived and landed in a clearing nearby, the medics rushed out and started treating his Daddy. They gave him drugs to help him cope with the pain.'

After they'd treated his Daddy they came and talked to Eddy. They wanted to know who had done the first aid. He told them it was him, under his Dad's instruction. They were sceptical at first.'

Eddy smiled in the trance.

'But as there was no other possible explanation, they accepted that it was Eddy after all.

They wanted to know what drugs he had given his father. So he was able to show them the bottle that he'd filled the syringe from.'

'I expect they were impressed?'

'Yes they were.'

This confirmed John's earlier theory. Eddy's treatment of his father was how he had been able to treat Marilyn so effectively.' John smiled to himself. 'Convenient and timely memory recall,' he thought.

Although it was too early to assess what the final outcome of Eddy's mental health issue would be, following his hypnotherapy, John felt pleased that his decision to treat Eddy this way had been right. He was pleased that he hadn't allowed himself to be swayed by the Professor's 'stone-age' view of hypnotherapy.

Here was proof that the sessions were working. He had tapped into Eddy's psyche in the right place at the right time.

Eddy continued commentating on his story.

'One of the helicopter medics came and spoke to him. Asked if he was injured.'

'And was he?'

'He only had a small bump on his head and bruises across his chest from the seatbelt.'

'He was lucky then, considering how badly his father was injured.'

'Yes, he was.'

'What happened when they'd released his Dad from the wreckage?'

'They carried him into the helicopter and Eddy ran over and held his hand. But his father must have gone to sleep because his hand was limp.

As they loaded the stretcher in, Eddy kissed his Dad's cheek.

As it was a small helicopter, at first they said Eddy couldn't go in it; that he would have to stay with the fire crew. He started to cry. He wanted to go with his Dad. But finally the doctor said they would squeeze him in somehow. Although he had to sit on his lap.

Pretty soon the helicopter took off while the medics were diligently monitoring his unconscious Dad's vital signs. Anyway after a noisy trip of about half an hour they landed at a hospital.

Did you know that helicopters have a big H to land on?' Eddy asked randomly.

'Yes, I've flown in helicopters before..'

'Eddy didn't. Anyway they took Daddy on a trolley into a room where Eddy couldn't go.

There were lots of people running round and a nurse came and checked Eddy over and gave him a drink, a sandwich and a bag of sweets.

When she'd finished looking after him she went and checked on his Daddy.

She came out from the room slowly, looking at him with sad eyes.

She started to speak, but Eddy knew something bad had happened and he ran past her into the room.

And there was nobody working on his Daddy but the sheet had been pulled up over his face. He shouted at her to take it off his Daddy's face.

But the nurse came and put her hands on Eddy's shoulders and knelt down and said she was very sorry but his Daddy was dead. She said everyone had done as much as they could to save him, but he had died.

Eddy said no you didn't. He'd kept his father alive and you have killed him. Eddy pulled the sheet off his Daddy's face and kissed him and told him that he loved him. And asked him to please wake up. He wants to go fishing with him again.

But his Daddy didn't move. After a while, the nurse put the sheet back over his Daddy's face again and took Eddy out of the room. Eddy started crying. He had been such a brave boy until then.'

The trace on the monitor had peaked, so John, with tears in his eyes, stopped the session and slowly brought Eddy out of the trance.

'Are you Ok Eddy?'

'Yes thank you,' he said, not showing any signs of remembering anything about his tragic story.

'I think we have done enough for today,' John said, surprisingly touched by Eddy's story. 'Please feel free to go when you want. We'll leave it now for a time before we have another session. You are doing really well,' he informed his patient.'

'Will you be doing all my treatments or are you working with the Professor on the trial that we are on?

'No I'll be doing all your sessions, but I might have to help the Professor from time to time. Why do you ask?'

'I was just wondering,' he lied, secretly pleased. Now he had some information to give back to the woman he knew as Sheila. 'She will be very pleased with me,' he thought. 'I think, I'll go now,' Eddy said, leaving.

'Yes Ok Eddy. Goodbye and well done again.'

Eddy left John's consulting room, thinking about his next move to get the other bits of information for Sheila.

Meanwhile John gazed out of the window deep in thought.

'Wow! Poor kid. No wonder he was traumatised,' John thought, feeling completely drained. He was surprised by the impact on his own emotions. The tragic ten year old's trauma had got to him.

His own ability to remain detached, cultivated over many years when listening to patient's, sometimes strange and harrowing stories, had been breached.

'Now I know the detail of his suffering, how do I take him to the next step and unlock the door to allow him some semblance of normality? That is the question.'

Chapter Forty-three

Eddy pondered about getting the information for his new friend while he was in the building with a legitimate reason. Was it too risky? Then again,' he argued, no one could tell him off.' Undecided, he wrestled with his conscience as he walked slowly down the stairs towards the exit.

Finally, Eddy made his mind up. He decided that he would take the opportunity to get the other information Sheila wanted after all.

'I expect she'll give me a kiss if I get it,' he thought excitedly.

He knew that the information was likely to be kept in the records office, but in order to get in there, he had to pass Laura's desk.

When he got down to the ground floor Laura wasn't at her desk, she was close by watering some house plants and had her back to him.

'Shall I chance it?' he wondered, stopping briefly. 'Yes. Marilyn would say be brave,' he encouraged himself.

Quickly, he crept past her desk and went silently into the records office. Unfortunately, the door hinge squeaked as he closed it behind him.

Laura heard the squeak and shouted. 'Hello, anyone there?'

No response. 'Oh it must be the wind blowing the door,' she concluded and carried on with her watering regime.

Meanwhile, Eddy's blood had turned to ice as he stood still and waited for her to come in to the room and tell him off.

But she didn't, so after a few minutes, he carried on, relieved that he wasn't going to be quickly ejected.

As he looked around, he was stunned by the large number of documents and shelves groaning under the weight of rows and rows of books.

'Oh heavens! I'm never going to find anything in here. Where do I even start?' he puzzled, looking around, bewildered and unsure of what he was looking for.

He studied the list that Sophie had written for him again.

'Right, I must find the surnames of the missing ones, Digger, Peter and Mathew,' he mused, looking at the mystifying row of document drums wondering where to start.

Nevertheless he busied himself looking around randomly and was fortunate that he stumbled upon three files in a tray labelled 'No longer required'.

'Ah, what's this he wondered, flicking open the first file labelled 'Lucas'. Ah here we are!' he smiled to himself. 'Just what I wanted. Digger Lucas's file.'

He took a pen out of his pocket and copied the surnames from the other files onto his list very carefully. 'Digger Lucas; Peter Thomas; Mathew Henry.' Feeling pleased that he had even had the forethought to bring a pen with him.

'Now what else did I have to find,' he wondered, checking his note. 'The name of the drugs, that's right,' he confirmed.

He thumbed through their records again and spotted the name of the drugs with which they all had been treated.

Eddy quickly copied the complicated name very carefully, fearful any minute that someone might come in and tell him off. *'Phenloramide its Trade name was Mandragal @ Scana-Landis Corp.'*

As he completed writing it down and had put the files back where he found them, Laura came into the room clutching more files. She was surprised to see him.

'Oh God you made me jump! Eddy, what are you doing in here anyway? You know it's off bounds to patients,' she berated.

'I...I...I've...ummm... come to the wrong room,' he pleaded. 'I've just had a session with Doctor John and got confused.'

'Well, I think you've been here long enough to know that this room is out of bounds,' she scolded. 'Good bye Eddy,' she said holding the door open.

'Sorry, Goodbye Laura,' he grovelled, leaving.

Despite being told off by Laura, Eddy departed happy that he now had the information that would make the woman he knew as Sheila, happy too.

Chapter Forty-four

John knocked on the Professor's closed door and waited to be invited in.

'Unusual,' he thought. 'He normally leaves his door open.'

After a few minutes, John heard the invitation.

'Come,' the Professor invited, clearly irritated by the interruption.

'Have you got a few minutes Professor?'

'No not really. But as you've disturbed me. What is it?' he said brusquely.

John was surprised at the irritation in the academics voice.

'Well just to add to your deliberations. I am moving out from the flat here in the hospital,' John informed the Professor.

'Why? It's convenient for the hospital to have you on the premises.'

'Well it might be convenient for the hospital, but it's not for me. I haven't done over a decade of training to be doing Junior doctor night time activities.' John said vehemently.

'I can't say that I am not disappointed. The nurses and junior doctors talk highly of you when they have called for your assistance,' the Professor admitted.

'Well now it's their turn to step up to the mark. Besides, I've a house viewing this afternoon and won't be around.'

'Well, I suppose I can't stop you,' the Professor reluctantly admitted.

'Incidentally, I had a strange conversation with Eddy at the culmination of my last session with him,' John advised the academic.

'I warned you about pursuing hypnotherapy. Well in his fragile mental state, why would you expect anything other than a strange conversation?' the other replied flippantly.

'May be, but for some reason he wanted to know if I was helping you on the trial.' John explained.

'Well you're not, are you?' the Professor said irritably.

'No, of course not. But something else odd happened, Laura found Eddy in the records office.'

'What the hell! What was he doing in there? He shouldn't have been in there,' the Professor said angrily.

'Yes I know and that's what Laura told him. She sent him off with a flea in his ear.'

'Was...did he touch anything?'

'Not that Laura could see. Why, is there something to hide in there?' the psychiatrist asked suspiciously.

'No of course not. But all the records are confidential. Laura will have to ensure that the door is locked from now on. We don't want any willy nilly characters wandering around in there,' the Professor insisted.

'Why would Eddy wander in there in the first place?' John wondered. 'In fact both Eddy and Marilyn are exhibiting strange behaviour There is something going on.'

'Strange behaviour! What do you mean?

'Well, according to the bus company, Marilyn decided she was an Aryan and didn't have to pay her bus fare. And Eddy threw hot chocolate drink in a woman's face.'

'As you know with our clients, these things happen from time to time. And your point is?'

'Do you think it's anything to do with the trial medication that they're on?'

'No, of course not,' the Professor said dismissively.

'Eddy tells me that all the others in the sheltered housing complex are on it too.'

'Yes that's right. Moving them to the complex was a sort of a bribe if you like. I needed to recruit some 'guinea pig' patients. It was fortunate that I could bring them together in that area. It makes administering the drug and monitoring the effects a lot easier.'

'So what is this trial all about?' John asked concerned.

'Oh, it's nothing really, just behavioural rationalisation and monitoring,' the Professor said, downplaying John's concern. 'It's something with which I'm experimenting.'

'So you have been giving this new drug to your clients?' John asked.

'Yes of course. You know, that occasionally you have to test these things out. Sometimes the benefits far outweigh the dangers. Sometimes you have to navigate between regulations to get anywhere.'

'Are you implying that you are conducting a clinical trial without getting it approved?' John asked. 'Surely this eminent Professor wouldn't put his career on the line and ignore regulations,' he thought.

'It is properly controlled of course,' the Professor explained. 'I am working with a top pharmaceuticals organisation to develop the drug. Look at the drug product paper,' the Professor invited, removing a document from his desk drawer, and offering it to John. 'You will see that I've been working with my friends at Scana-Landis to develop and refine it.'

Chapter Forty-five

John studied the detailed product paper, which seemed to concur with the Professors explanation. It had all the appropriate classifications associated with any drug. Including its name ***Phenloramide*** and trade name '*Mandragal @ Scana-Landis Corp.*

John handed the document back to the academic.

'Very professional but what is it supposed to do?'

'Acts to suppress the abnormal brain activity seen in seizure by reducing electrical conductance among brain cells by stabilizing the inactive state of voltage-gated sodium channels.'

'Sounds adventurous,' John observed.

'We have developed Phenloramide for the treatment and prevention of Grand mal, petit mal (absence seizures) and temporal lobe epilepsy.

Mood swings are reduced in patients with bipolar affective disorder.

Its anxiolytic properties can be used to control generalised anxiety disorder.

Its synaptic activity raises the pain gate threshold making it useful to control neurogenic pain associated with trigeminal neuralgia, sciatica and in terminal care.

As I say, it's in the early days for the drug yet. But I'm also looking at DNA implications too.'

'DNA?'

'Yes, it's just becoming clear how this reasonably new discovery can be used in medical science. It's full name is Deoxyribonucleic acid.'

'Yes, that's right. I've recently read about it in a medical journal. DNA is the chemical name for the molecule that carries genetic instructions in all living things isn't it?' John queried.

'Yes, 'It's the building block of life,' the Professor explained. 'Just like a cipher code.

'I believe the nucleotide bases of the DNA code are Adenine (A), 'Cytosine (C), Guanine (G), and Thymine (T),' John suggested.

'Top of the class. Yes that's right,' the Professor confirmed enthusiastically. 'Nice to see that you are keeping up with advances in medicine.'

'I pride myself in keeping abreast with all medical developments,' John explained. 'The science is exciting and ever changing.'

'It's quite exciting to imagine what will eventually come from this discovery of DNA over the coming years,' the academic continued, beaming.

'And you are saying that this will help your research?' John wondered.

'Oh yes, most definitely. It's the chemical balance that I'm interested in. If we can find the right drug to rebalance the DNA in the brain, then I think we can cure Mental health problems,' the Professor enthused. 'Unfortunately, the science community aren't yet ready for this type of innovative thinking.'

'Surely the psychiatry world will pounce on your work?'

'No, not yet. I need to keep it quiet until I have developed the theory sufficiently and I have written my scientific paper.'

'Your secret's safe with me,' John confirmed. 'But is it working?' John queried.

'It's early days yet and we are still refining it. As I say, I am working with Scana-Landis to modify it and to obtain the correct balance.'

'Why are you developing it along these lines?' John asked.

'As I've said before. I believe that all mental health problems stem from the same cause.'

'Yes, I remember you saying that. But what proof have you got?' John questioned, sceptically.

'I'm working on it. If we can unravel that, then I think we can cure ALL mental health issues before they even manifest themselves.'

'Sounds like Utopia,' John said sceptically.

'That's what I'm aiming for,' the Professor said optimistically. 'Don't fail to undertake a challenge because it's hard,' he counselled.

'How many people have you treated with this drug?' John probed.

'I…I err.. can't remember off hand. It's in my records,' the Professor said evasively. 'But obviously it's a relatively small number at this stage of development.'

'So are you treating Eddy Jones with this?'

'Yes. Eddy was one of the first on the trial. I was encouraged by the changes in him…to start off with. But then things seemed to go awry as the cumulative effect of the Phenloramide built up.'

'So your drugs could have been causing some damage then!'

'Conceivably. But that's what trials are all about. However, it's still in the alpha stage, shall we say it's still informal at the moment.'

'Still in the alpha stage! Surely you have got authority to trial?'

'I'm currently processing the documentation,' the Professor revealed reluctantly. 'So many of my ideas have been hijacked because of bureaucracy getting in the way. No, I'm keeping this quiet until I'm ready.'

'I wish you hadn't told me that. You place me with a very difficult dilemma. Oh. I don't know what to say.' John said, starting to pace the office. 'Should I inform the Medical Council and…'

'Don't take that attitude with me. It's all recorded properly,' the Professor said defensively, collapsing onto his chair. It was as if John's observations had caused his energy to dissipate and he was completely deflated.

'I'm sorry, but ethically I am in the horns of a dilemma. I must voice my concerns otherwise I could be implicated in bad practice as I work here,' John explained awkwardly.

'You'll have to be quick. I believe that we have already had the media sniffing around to try to discredit my work,' the Professor revealed.

'Oh, that's not good.'

'Unfortunately three of the patients on my trial died. Not through my drug treatment I must add,' the Professor added quickly. 'One was stabbed and the other two were riddled with disease from years of previous chemical abuse, before they even came here. But they all had to have an autopsy.'

'Well if it wasn't a Phenloramide related death, surely you have no worries.'

'Unfortunately, the pathologist who conducted the autopsy was very thorough and when he examined the victim's, he found considerable damage.'

'Brain damage?'

'Yes, he found that in all three of them there was a part of the brain missing.'

'A what?' John gasped, unsure of what he'd heard..

'There was a hole in the frontal lobe,' the Professor revealed dramatically.

'Significant then?' John observed, as an understatement.

'I believe the pathologist subsequently sent samples to a forensic neuropathologist. Who found trace elements of Phenloramide, the drug that I had been prescribing to them.

'Oh dear.'

'Although there is no proof that Phenloramide was the cause of death. The extent of the brain damage is concerning,' the Professor revealed. 'Somehow it has got to the media and I am now also being targeted by the Anti Mental Health care brigade.'

'Targeted? How?'

'Stalking, graffiti on my car. My wife has just telephoned and said that we have a group of noisy protesters outside my house.'

'Sorry to hear that,' John said. 'So that's why he is grumpy,' he realised

'It's one of the risks that we, as pioneers, take in order to move science forward. We have to take bold steps and dare to dream, the Professor said passionately. 'Well if there's nothing else. I've got work to do,' he said abruptly.

'No nothing else,' John said feeling guilty at adding to the academics worries.

'John, I should think long and hard about what you do with that information that I've just given you,' the Professor warned.

John left, now perplexed about his options.

Chapter Forty-six

John made his way downstairs to Laura's desk and was pleased to see her there.

'Ah, just the lady I wanted to speak to.'

'I've very rarely been called a lady,' she replied, smiling.

'I just wanted to say thank you for the tip off about the housing agent.'

'Any luck?'

'Yes, I'm looking at an apartment this afternoon on the East Esplanade.'

'East Esplanade! lovely. That's where all the business professionals live,' she informed him. 'You'll be in good company there with the solicitors, eminent surgeons, Judges, and airline pilots, to name just a few.'

'Perhaps I can even find some wealthy clients from that lot then,' he joked.

'Well, let me know how you get on and if I can help you at all?'

'I was hoping you'd offer. Thanks.'

'My pleasure.'

'On a business front. I've just had a lengthy chat with the Professor. Laura, I'm a bit concerned about what he's doing with those patients in the sheltered housing,' John admitted.

'What do you mean?'

'I think that he's using the residents as guinea pigs and is in collusion with the drug company in developing a new form of unlicensed medication,' he revealed. 'He showed me the drug pamphlet.'

'Yes well that's what he does. He is constantly researching new ways to tackle mental illnesses, admitted Laura defensively.'

'I know, but the drugs he is giving the trial patients appear to suppress their emotions, cause hallucinations and worse.'

'What do you mean worse?'

'Possibly cause brain damage,' John said, dramatically.

'Why do you say that?' she puzzled. 'What proof have you got?'

'He told me about the pathologists finding holes in the brains of former residents who were on his trial.'

'The Professor is an eminent scientist, he wouldn't do anything like that to deliberately endanger people's lives, surely?' Laura wondered, now unsure of the certainty of her views.

'No I agree, he wouldn't do that deliberately. But the growing protests around the world claim that our current methods for treating mental health are cruel and brutal. They irrationally compare it to the ancient habit of burning witches.' John observed.

'Oh that's a nonsense. We are trying to treat them, to make them better,' Laura retorted passionately.

'Ok, if the Professor has nothing to hide why doesn't Eddy's file have records of his current medication regime?' he challenged.

'Perhaps it's misfiled,' she suggested, cautiously.

'I confronted the Professor about it and he became very defensive.'

'I can understand that if you are questioning his professionalism,' Laura countered. 'Yes Ok, but even if you're right, what's the alternative?'

'The alternative to damaging brains? Well it's to find better ways of putting our clients back into society,' John said avidly.

'But you have already seen what reaction we get from the locals even with the current medication,' Laura countered.

'Ok with our clients emotional differences, I accept that there will be some problems. But it has to be better than the chemical cosh that the Professor is subduing them with?' There has to be a better way, surely?' John said, passionately.

'On the other hand, I've been to the meetings where the locals demand that we chemically handcuff our patients,' Laura amplified.

'Why?'

'So they claim, that they can live their lives in the knowledge that our charges aren't going to be a danger to their families,' Laura explained.

'I suppose they're right. There is no short term fix. Researchers have been looking for the cause of mental health issues for a long time…and the best thing we can do is to do what society expects of us, I suppose…..just manage the problem,' John said resignedly. 'But there has to be another way and I hope to prove that with my hypnotherapy treatments.'

Chapter Forty-seven

John was mesmerised by the lovely three bedroom apartment that he was viewing. It was the most positive he'd felt for a long time. It was a dream home.

'What a magnificent place,' he'd enthused to the agent. 'I need to pinch myself. I've always wanted to live by the sea and here I am. Sea, sky and beach.'

Without hesitation, he agreed to buy the one million dollar dream residence on the lavish East Esplanade in the suburb of Manly.

The apartment was located just metres from Manly Beach, with its cafes, restaurants, and other beach amenities and had magnificent harbour views.

He couldn't wait to share his good news with Laura. So at the end of the viewing he hurried back to tell her.

She looked up as he rushed into reception.

'Well it looks like the cat has found the cream,' she smiled.

'Yes. You should see this place, it's absolutely fantastic,' John gushed, like a kid excitedly describing a Christmas present. 'Here look at the brochure, he said thrusting it under her nose.

Laura studied the creased Real Estate pamphlet, *'The stunning French style apartment boasted timeless appeal, charm and convenience.*

It has spacious interiors, brightly lit, accentuated by large French windows and 13-foot shadow edge ceilings, highlighting its 1908 heritage, yet with a contemporary design.

Just steps to Manly Village, it is perfectly placed to enjoy local world-famous beaches, cosmopolitan eateries, and a vibrant social scene right at Manly Wharf.

'Oh that sounds lovely. I can't wait to see it,' she enthused, buoyed by John's excitement. 'Tell you what, it's my lunch break shortly. Why don't we go and have a look,' Laura suggested.

'Ok, I'll ring the agent and get him to meet us there,' John agreed.

They met the agent outside the apartment block and rode the lift together to the top floor. The agent opened the door for Laura to enter first.

Like John, she was overwhelmed by the lovely apartment with its magnificent views.

It was indeed what he was looking for. With a large open-plan living area, which opened up on to an entertainers size balcony with magnificent sea views and featuring a large area for a barbecue.

It's master bedroom opened up on to the balcony and gave incredible views.

It had a new designer kitchen, complete with gas stove, dishwasher, stone benches and white subway tiled splashback's.

The bathroom was fitted with a frameless shower and a separate designer bath.

The large bedrooms, were delightfully appointed including built-In Wardrobes.

The fact that it was located on the top floor of the apartment block was not a problem because it had lift access. It also came with a garage nearby for the new BMW that he had recently purchased.

'Oh John, this is absolutely lovely,' Laura agreed, as they wandered around the apartment.

'Yes, I'm looking forward to moving in as soon as possible,' he said, beaming from ear to ear.

Chapter Forty-eight

John couldn't wait to leave the hospital flat. Fortunately, the sale for his new apartment went through very quickly. And with Laura's assistance he moved in within a couple of weeks of the viewing.

'Well here you are in your new apartment,' Laura said finally shutting the door after the last delivery man had left.'

'Brilliant isn't it? It went pretty smoothly I thought, John said, looking around.

'I don't know about you but after a hectic and very long day, I'm shattered,' Laura confessed, slumping down on the newly arrived settee.

'I can't understand why, I mean all you've done all day is erect curtains,' John joked.

'And what about the early start, buying all the various goods for the kitchen and then stocking the fridge and cupboards with provisions,' she said testily.

'Oh Ok, I'll give you that. But what about those poor delivery people humping stuff up here to the top floor? Just as well that I didn't have anything major to move from the hospital flat though,' John observed.

'They must have been shattered. I hope you gave them a big tip, ' Laura asked.'

'The guys were only doing their job,' he observed... but, yes I did,' he confessed.

'They certainly earned it.'

'Oh! while you were out, the telephone people came and fitted your posh new phone too,' Laura explained. 'It's got lots of buttons on it.'

'Oh has it? I'll probably never use them. Technology leaves me cold,' he confessed. 'However food is something that I'm good at,' he boasted. ' I'll cook a barbie for you on our new barbeque out on the veranda,' John proposed. 'How does that sound?'

'Great, but I could do with a drink first,' she added.

'Ok, no problem, as you know the fridge is newly stocked with our favourite wine,' he said opening the door and selecting a bottle. 'Now where did I put the wine glasses,' he asked looking around.

'Under your nose, on the sideboard,' she pointed out.

'Oh, yes.'

John poured two generous glasses of chilled wine and handed one to Laura.

'Thank you for all your help and your 20 x 20 vision with the wine glasses,' he joked.

'My pleasure. Here's to your new freedom away from the hospital,' she proposed.

'Cheers,' they said in unison, chinking glasses.

'Umm, this is nice,' she cooed, as she sipped her wine.

'Yes, it's the same one that I had when we went to Surfers Pavilion that first time, when you seduced me,' he said, fluttering his eyelids coquettishly.

'I never did,' she protested, smiling. 'You took advantage of me. I only showed you the sights.'

'And I've loved seeing those sights ever since,' he said saucily.

'Cheeky!' Laura replied demurely.

John cooked a delicious BBQ and afterwards, as the wine flowed John cosied up to Laura. 'Thank you for helping me. It needed a woman's gentle touch to bring the place to life. And now, how would you like a man's touch to complete your day?' he said seductively.

'What are you suggesting kind sir?' she said lustily.

'Well, as I don't know a lot of people here yet, this first barbie was my house warming, with the most important people in attendance.'

'Yes, I'd agree,' she said.

'And now we move inside to the master bedroom,' he said. 'For the bed warming.'

Gently he lifted her out of her chair and carried her effortlessly into the huge, newly furnished bedroom.

Chapter Forty-nine

The following morning, Laura woke to find an empty space beside her. She slipped on one of John's shirts, which looked like a nightdress on her slim figure, and she wandered around the apartment looking for him.

'Ah, there you are John,' Laura said, finding him in the lounge in front of a computer. 'What are you doing peering at that screen? You're not working again are you?'

'No. I'm doing a family history search. I bought a disc off one of these Genealogical firms. He took his eyes from the screen and looked at her as she walked towards him.

'My, you look very sexy in my shirt. You wear it a lot better than I do, although it's a bit big on your beautiful body. Perhaps I ought to remove it?'

'No it's Ok, thank you. I shall maintain my modesty and keep it on. Anyway, I didn't think that you were interested in finding out where your roots were.'

'I've changed my mind. I was talking to an 80 year old patient just before he died ... and he was saying how awful it was to die without any of his family around him, and....'

'You're not thinking of dying just yet are you?' Laura interrupted. 'Otherwise I shall have to find myself a new man.'

'No, of course not. But it got me thinking...you know about things... and well I think it would be nice to see if....I...'

'What? If there's an inheritance waiting for you?... You never know you might be a millionaire. Perhaps I'll forget about looking for another man, I think I'll stay with you.' Laura smiled, giving him a kiss on the top of his head.

'Yeah that would be nice. Unfortunately, the chances of me finding any family history, let alone an inheritance is probably a million to one,' John suggested, realistically.

'Yeah, but if you don't look, you won't find anyway I guess,' she added.

'Oh very profound.'

'What about birth certificates?' Laura asked.

'Haven't got one. Mum wasn't good with her paperwork,' John explained.

'What about your dad?'

'I don't know who he was. Mum brought me up by herself. I think Dad died, but I don't know. In our house. talk of him was forbidden,' he revealed.'

'Oh, how terrible. I can't imagine life without my father. We used to have good fun together winding my mother up.'

'You are lucky to have had time with him,' John pointed out. '

'Don't you feel a sense of loss?' Laura said, profoundly.

'You don't miss what you never had,' John responded quietly.

'Oh that's terrible,' Laura acknowledged.

'Nothing that I can do about it though. But I often wondered what it would have been like to have had him around,' John said reflectively.

'Obviously, you've got some dark secret in your closet then,' she giggled.

'Come here and I'll show you something else in my closet,' he said suggestively.

'Oh. You're just a dirty old man,' Laura said, coquettishly standing next to him.

'Here, that button's coming undone,' he pointed at the top of his shirt

'No it isn't,' she said, looking at where he was pointing.

'Oh yes it is,' he said standing, 'Because I've just decided.' Give me a kiss…fortune hunter,' John teased. Kissing her deeply.

As they kissed, he slowly undid all the buttons of the shirt and slipped it off her shoulders on to the floor, at their feet.

Chapter Fifty

At an office in the television production centre, Sophie was plotting the key milestones for her documentary about the Professor and the Imagine Institute, when she spotted an interesting newspaper article.

She re-read the article again, making notes as she digested the facts.

Patient refuses treatment

Court of Appeal backs the case of a mentally ill, brilliant, scientist who is refusing to receive treatment.

Professor Stephen Yung has successfully appealed against his medical carers to, as he calls it, suppress his intellect by prescribing him mind altering drugs. Professor Yung started showing signs of mental illness in his early 20s. In between bouts of ill health he wrote some brilliant treaties on the development of the developing world. It was during the delivery of a thesis on the dynamics of the human psyche that he first was seen to become ill. 'Brilliance is on the borders of insanity.' he is credited in saying.

'I wonder how many other mental health patients feel the same? It might form a good talking point for my documentary,' she thought.

'Brilliance is on the borders of insanity!' She re-read the phrase.'. 'Well I reckon if that's right, then there are a lot of 'brilliant' people around that Institute's sheltered accommodation,' she laughed mockingly.

'I wonder if I can persuade my stooge, Eddy, to refuse to take his medication and see what the Professor does then?"

Later that day, wearing her Sheila disguise, Sophie met Eddy, at the agreed time, on the park bench near his house.

'So Eddy, have you got the answers to the three questions that I gave you?' she asked, fully expecting a negative report.

'Yes, I have the information, here,' he said, proudly digging out the piece of paper that she'd given him, now containing his notes.

'Here,' he said, giving it to her.

'Oh well done,' she praised, for his unexpected success.

'I had to write it down,' he explained. 'But my handwriting isn't very good.'

'You can say that again,' she said, looking at the scrawl on the note. 'What does this say?' she demanded pointing at his scribbled entry.

'It's the surnames you wanted; this is Digger Lucas; Peter Thomas; Mathew Henry,' he said, running his finger around his writing.

'If you say so,' she said coldly. 'But more importantly, what was the drug they were all taking?'

'There, on the paper,' he said, turning the note over. 'I printed it because it was a hard word.'

Sophie read his scruffy print. 'Phenloramide its Trade name was Mandragal @ Scana-Landis Corp.' 'Are you sure?' she questioned.

'Yes, I think so. I wrote it down from their records,' he revealed.

'This is great. Well done. And now finally, is your psychiatrist working with the Professor?'

'He says he might have to,' Eddy revealed.

'Might have to, I suppose that will have to do. Ok, thank you Eddy. You have done a brilliant job,' she gushed, hugging him and kissing him on the cheek.

Eddy was taken aback by her unexpected embrace and put his hand on his cheek where she'd kissed him. But his euphoria wasn't to last long, as suddenly there was a lot of shouting nearby.

Chapter Fifty-one

'Eddy, listen. What's all that noise?' Sophie asked.

'I don't know Sheila,' he said, using her pseudonym.

'It sounds like there's a fight going on,' she announced.

'Oh God,' Eddy uttered nervously.

'Let's go and see what's going on,' Sophie said excitedly. Fuelled by her journalistic sense of chasing a news story, she was often at the forefront of incidents, often violent protests.

'No I'll go.. go and go home,' Eddy muttered, stepping back.

'You're scared,' Sophie concluded, deriding Eddy's nervousness.

'No, it's…It's just…it's just that violence upsets me. The thought of someone deliberately hurting someone else I find terrible. I'll see you later,' Eddy said, starting to leave for home.

'Ok, if you're scared, it's the best place,' Sophie said, disparagingly.

Sophie ran to the source of the shouting several streets away, leaving a frightened Eddy behind.

When Sophie arrived she encountered a small baying crowd of fifteen people egging on a woman who was fighting a man.

The pair were on the ground trading punches. Despite his intention of running away, Eddy had eventually worked up enough courage and talked himself into following nervously behind Sophie.

'God it's a woman!' Sophie declared. 'I wonder what it's all about?' she said to no one in particular.

'Oh, the scruffy git was mistreating his dog, so the woman laid into him,' one of the crowd informed her.

'She's doing alright too. Look she's given him a bloody nose,' Sophie observed. 'And a black eye too, by the look of it.'

'Marilyn. Oh my god it's Marilyn,' Eddy discovered as he got closer. 'What is she doing? I must help her,' he said, overcoming his fear and starting to go towards the brawling couple.

'Hang on Eddy. Here come the police. Don't get mixed up in it,' Sophie counselled, grabbing his arm and holding him back.

The crowd parted as the Police Sergeant arrived and took charge.

'All right let's break it up then,' Jon Baldy called, grabbing hold of Marilyn's arm as she was just about to land another punch. 'Oh it's you again,' he said, recognising her. 'I should have guessed you'd be at the centre of it.'

'Get her off me,' her desperate and blooded opponent shouted.

The Policeman lifted a struggling Marilyn off her opponent and with great difficulty dragged her away from him.

'I haven't finished with him yet,' Marilyn said, kicking out and struggling to break the Policeman's hold. 'He was mistreating his dog. I'll give him, hurting a defenceless animal.'

'Get the mad bitch off me. She's a bleeding nutter,' the man screeched, scrabbling away from her crablike on his back, whilst also maintaining eye contact with his opponent

'Alright that will do,' the Policeman said, tightening his grip on the still struggling woman. 'What's this all about?'

'He was being cruel to his dog. I saw him kick it,' Marilyn screeched. 'He doesn't deserve to have a dog. You should take it off him if he can't treat it right.'

'Where's the dog now?' the Policeman asked looking around.

'He ran off as soon as they started fighting,' one of the crowd informed him.

'Marilyn are you alright?' Eddy asked anxiously, rushing over to her.

'What are you doing here Eddy? Come to show off your new girlfriend?' Marilyn accused disapprovingly, after spotting Sophie with him.

'No, not at all. I was a bit concerned about you, that was all. Are you Ok? He asked sympathetically.'

'Not that you care anyway,' she said, spitting blood from her split lip onto the pavement at his feet.

'Right you two,' the Police Sergeant addressed the two protagonists. 'I don't want any more of this fighting from either of you. And Marilyn, if I see any more hassle from you, you'll be in prison before you know it. Do you understand?'

"Living in that place, feels like we're already there anyway,' she muttered under her breath.

Sophie noted Marilyn's muttered observation and mentally added it to the script for her documentary.

'Do you understand, what I'm saying?' the Policeman repeated firmly.

''Yes I suppose so,' she accepted reluctantly.

'Now on your way. And you, if I hear about you mistreating that dog again I shall run you in so fast your feet won't touch the ground. Do you understand?' he told the blooded dog owner.

'Yeth,' the other said through his split lip.

'Now clear off, all of you. Or I'll nick you all for a breach of the peace,' he told the crowd.

As they walked away from the scene of the fight Sophie quizzed Eddy. 'That woman, is she your girlfriend?'

'Yes, she was, but you're my girlfriend now aren't you?' Eddy said watching Marilyn limping away.

'If you say so Eddy. If you say so,' Sophie said, unconvincingly.

Chapter Fifty-two

Eddy knocked on the consulting room door.

'Come in,' John's voice from inside commanded.

Eddy did as he was bid and entered the now familiar room.

'Hello Eddy, I hope that you were Ok after the last session and it wasn't too draining on you,' the hypnotherapist said.

'I did feel a little tired. But it was Ok, thanks.'

'Understandable, it was a very intense session, but we are getting to the bottom of your problems now..'

'Ok,' Eddy said meekly.

'I'm very pleased with progress. Today, we'll strip back some more layers,' John enthused.

As before, John put Eddy in a trance, suitably wired up with the EEG cap.

'I want you to relax, let all the tensions of your day go, listen to my voice, relax...relax. You feel light. You can drift to sleep. Remember you are Eddy's observer, so nothing can hurt you.'

Eddy was quickly in a trance and John took him back to his experiences of the crash.

'Remember that after the long agonising wait to be rescued, the firemen arrived and Eddy and his father were flown to hospital in a helicopter,' John reminded him.'

'Yes he remembers,' Eddy confirmed.

'Then the nurse checked Eddy over to make sure that he didn't have any injuries, does he remember that too?'

'Yes he does.'

'What happened next?'

'They wouldn't let him see his dad again. After many hours waiting his step mother came to the hospital room. She was very, very upset,' Eddy explained.

'I expect that she was.'

'She wouldn't believe that her husband was dead. She kept crying very loudly, and saying it wasn't true.'

'What did she say to Eddy?'

'She had been frantically worrying about them both. They were only supposed to be going to camp for one night and then home the second night.'

'Understandable. 'So what did she do?'

'She reported them missing to the Police.'

'What did the Police do?'

'Nothing. She couldn't persuade the police to search for them. They convinced her that Eddy and his father were probably just staying over for another night.

Then the following day she heard that there was a big fire where they were proposing to go camping, so she rang them again.

But the Police said everybody had been evacuated from the area of the fire and they were probably in a refuge centre somewhere,' Eddy explained.

'That must have been horrible for her then to find that they weren't safe after all?' John suggested.

'Yes it was. The call from the hospital to say that there had been an accident was a big shock to her. Especially after being reassured by the Police that they were safe,' Eddy said dramatically.

'Yes I can understand that. She would have been terribly shocked.'

'But when the news of the crash came out, the Police drove her all the way from Sydney in a fast car to the hospital to see her step son.'

'I expect, when she arrived at the hospital, she was relieved to see that at least Eddy wasn't hurt?

'No, not really. They didn't have that close a relationship. Actually I don't think she liked him at all,' Eddy revealed.'

'Poor kid,' John thought. After all the trauma that he had been through, especially losing his father in such an awful way, a hug would have been so powerful to comfort him.'

'She became hysterical and blamed everybody for her husband's death, the firemen, the doctors, the hospital but mainly Eddy.'

'During trauma like that it often happens. They don't actually mean to blame anyone, it's just an irrational reaction to devastating and incomprehensible news,' John explained.

'But her accusations made Eddy feel very guilty. He questioned himself. In spite of the paramedics and nurses compliments about how well he had medically treated his father. Eddy wondered whether he had really done enough to save him. Was there something he had missed?'

'Eddy shouldn't have burdened himself with it. He was only a child and he did more than any other child of his age could have done. Against all the odds, Eddy actually preserved his father's life until they were rescued,' John encouraged.

'He did, didn't he? Eddy reluctantly agreed.

'It's more likely that his father died because of his major crush injuries,' John observed.

'What do you mean?'

'Well, what often happens in this type of accident, as soon as casualties are removed from crashed vehicles, victims sometimes 'bleed out' because the compression of blood vessels is then removed.

Nothing anyone could have done, least of all Eddy, would have been able to save his father,' John reassured him. 'And remember while he was in Eddy's care he was alive until the adults took over.'

'But it wasn't enough. He died,' Eddy said woefully.

'So here is the root of the problem,' John thought. 'This is the cause of Eddy's mental health issues. Guilt! Guilt from his step mother's accusations. Guilt from his own perception. All this on top of the trauma of the accident. Coupled with childhood bereavement of his much loved father. No wonder the kid had problems.'

Chapter Fifty-three

John moved the conversation on, and away from the death of Eddy's father.

'So did Eddy come home from hospital with his step mother?'

'Yes, but she was in a bad place. She loved his father. Her husband did everything for her. She was totally lost without him. In spite of the lack of their emotional closeness, Eddy had to support her, like his Dad had instructed him.'

'But he was a ten year old kid. He was grieving too.'

'Yes but his Dad had tasked him with this important job. While they were waiting to be rescued, he had told Eddy that If anything happened to him, Eddy had to be brave and support his step mum and carry on with the career plans that they had mapped out for Eddy.'

'Old before his time,' John thought. 'How did Eddy cope at his father's funeral?'

'As he had promised his Dad, he had to be strong for his step-mother. She was very, very upset and some of the adults had to support her too. So although he wanted to cry, he stopped himself.'

'And after the funeral?'

'His step mother went straight to bed, the Doctor prescribed her with some tablets.'

'And what about Eddy?

'He went to his favourite place, the tree house that his Daddy had built for him. And he stared at his favourite picture.'

'What was the picture?' John enquired.

'It was a photo that his Daddy had taken of him holding a large 16lb trout that he had caught. It was on one of their last fishing trips together.'

'Did that make him sad?'

'Yes, but as he'd promised his Dad that he would be brave, he didn't cry.'

'Sometimes it's best to cry, to let out sadness. Especially as it was such a big loss for Eddy. He was a very brave young child.'

'Eddy was always with his dad when he wasn't working. They would spend a lot of time together. And now he had nothing to look forward to. Only the black uncertain future.'

A tear ran down Eddy's cheek.

'Dad reckoned that Eddy could talk to 'grown ups' in their own 'language'. He knew a lot of things about grown up topics.

His Dad helped him achieve a lot of things. He was patient, kind and very clever. His Dad taught him to do first aid to a high level, often practising his bandaging techniques on his toys, pets and friends.'

'Hence that's how you tended to your dad and Marilyn by using your first aid training?' John thought.

'Eddy was going to be a doctor when he grew up. Just like his Dad.'

John recalled the ferry discussion with Eddy and understood where Eddy had the idea of becoming a doctor. It was a seed planted when he was a kid. The career plan, of course! That never happened.

'The senior citizens liked him. They said that he didn't have an ounce of bad in him; said he was a good kid …. had bright, keen eyes, a ready smile and acres of self-confidence,' Eddy continued reflectively.

'So what happened to his step mother?' John asked.

'She never got over her husband's death. I think she went back to the UK.'

'So when did Eddy come back to Australia?'

'He didn't leave. She left him here. She left without him.'

'She did what? But she was his mother!'

'Step mother,' Eddy corrected. 'She really didn't like him anyway. She called him an arrogant little shit. Said that he was old before his time. Said he was a miniature version of his father….said he even spoke with the same mannerisms. She couldn't bear being reminded of her loss… Because Eddy tried to emulate his father in his promised role of looking after her, she reckoned that Eddy talked down to her.'

'Mmm, she was probably right. I wouldn't want a precocious ten year old talking down to me either,' John thought.

'Shortly after, she disowned Eddy. She said that he become even more difficult to control after his father's death. Told the authorities that she had tried to control him for a couple of years but eventually gave up and decided to go back to the UK.'

'Without you?' 'Heartless cow,' John thought.

'Eddy said that he wouldn't go with her anyway, even if she wanted him to, which she didn't. Especially as he visited his father's grave regularly and talked to him.

So she left Eddy with the parents of one of his friends from the doctors practice.

But that didn't work, he went into complete withdrawal.'

'Post-Traumatic Stress had caught up with him, I expect.' John surmised. 'Because Eddy kept it at bay by storing up his grief rather than letting it go. It was like a pressure cooker. It was going to come out at some time.'

'Eventually Eddy was put up for adoption in a home. It was awful. He ran away several times. He really hated it.'

'I can understand that. It's all starting to make sense now. Poor kid he suffered trauma upon trauma,' John concluded.

'Then they fostered him out. But although the foster folk were nice, they were strict disciplinarians, he couldn't fit in with their family and they punished him with a leather belt. So eventually they sent him back to the orphanage.'

'From pillar to post, poor soul.'

'The orphanage was actually a home for unwanted kids. Again he didn't fit in there either. The other kids said he was too posh and 'up himself'. He got bullied and beaten up several times.'

'Poor kid.'

'So eventually he ended up in a hospital for disturbed children.'

'An asylum? Oh how awful. Totally the wrong place. He just wanted someone to care for him, not lock him up,' John thought, frustrated that society allowed this dreadful episode to occur.

'They gave Eddy pills to sedate him and he became…a 'model patient.'

'A zombie, more like,' John muttered under his breath.

Chapter Fifty-four

'OK, you are no longer Eddy's observer. You are yourself again. Before I wake you up? Is there anything else on your mind that is bothering you?' the hypnotherapist asked.

'I have a secret but I must not tell the Doctor or the Professor,' Eddy muttered.

'What must you not tell them?' John queried, intrigued by Eddy's comment.

'You mustn't tell anybody, but I have to tell her about the Doctor and the Professor.'

'About the two of them? What about them?' John said enthralled.

'If the Doctor is working with the Professor on the trial,' Eddy relayed.

'Who has told you not to tell?'.

'Sheila has told me,' Eddy revealed.

'Sheila! Who is Sheila?'

'The Protest lady. The one who looked after me when I was knocked out,' Eddy explained.

'Why would she want to know that,' John puzzled. '

Alarm bells started ringing in John's head. 'Why would a protester want to know about them. Perhaps she is one of the activists demonstrating outside the Professors house,' he wondered.

'Why does she want to know?'

'I mustn't tell you. But I think it's for an award,' Eddy said conspiratorially, repeating the lie that Sophie had told him originally.

'An award! What sort of award? I wonder if that's a smoke screen. Perhaps it's actually that TV reporter that was after an interview with the Professor?' John pondered.

'Listen Eddy, you're not to tell her anything about the hospital, do you understand?' John directed, hoping that whilst he was still hypnotised, Eddy's sub conscious would remember the instruction. Little realising that it was already too late. Eddy had already passed sensitive information to the investigative reporter.

Finally, John decided to call an end to the session.

'Ok enough for today,' he said, bringing Eddy out of the trance. 'That was very fulfilling Eddy. How do you feel?'

'Very tired,' Eddy said, sitting up and swivelling his feet onto the floor.

'I'm not surprised. That was a very heavy session. Just sit there for a minute.' John instructed. 'Tell me what you know about Sheila?'

'Sheila?' Eddy puzzled.

'Yes the lady that came to your rescue after you were knocked over by that thug.,' John prompted.

'Oh yes of course, Sheila. She is very nice to me.

'So have you seen a lot of Sheila?' John probed.

'Yes we met in the café and on a bench and...' Someone threw a drink in her face and tried to blame me. But I didn't do it Doctor,' he pleaded.

'Obviously, another side effect of this dreaded medication,' John thought.

'But she still likes me anyway. She gave me a kiss. She's my new girlfriend,' Eddy smiled.

'Oh that's interesting, John thought. 'What is she up to, I wonder?'

'And what does Marilyn think about that?' the psychiatrist asked.

'She…she is jealous. She doesn't like her. But Marilyn is always fighting. I don't like that,' Eddy revealed.

'Perhaps it's because she is looking after you Eddy. Just be careful with this Sheila. She might not be what you think. I would hate to see you hurt.'

Chapter Fifty-five

Sophie smiled to herself, the evidence against the Professor and his dubious practices was stacking up nicely. But there were still some gaps in a rock solid case before she could finally seal the deal with the producer.

She had the names of the three former deceased patients, indications from her police contact about the autopsy results and the link with the drug, the possible collusion between the Institute's head doctors, the name of the drug and the pharmaceutical company.

'Now let's see what else that brainless Eddy can find out for me,' she thought.

Aware of Marilyn's dislike of her, she briefly met Eddy near his home and proposed that they went to the café.

'G'day, Eddy nice to see you,' she lied.

'It's nice to see you too,' he said genuinely, feeling excited.

'But I don't think that Marilyn likes me very much, so let's go to the café again. I'll buy.'

'OK, he agreed.

But Marilyn had already spotted their meeting and was tamping mad.

As they made their way to the café, Sophie explained the reason for meeting him again so soon.

'I need you to find out some more information about the Institute for me,' Sophie asked.

'Is it for the award?'

'Award?' she wondered, having forgotten about the lie to Eddy earlier.

'Yes you know. For the doctor and Professor,' he reminded her.

'Oh, oh yes, that's right. The award,' she backpedalled at her forgetfulness.

'I…I can't. I don't think that I'm allowed,' Eddy told her, subconsciously remembering John's caution not to tell her anything else.

'Why is that?' she queried, taken aback at his reluctance. 'I thought we were friends?'

'Yes we are. You're my girlfriend aren't you?' Eddy sought to reconfirm their relationship.

'Yes, if you say so,' she smirked. 'But friends tell each other things, such as secrets don't they?' she pointed out.

'Yes. I suppose. But I can't say anything about the Institute. Doctor John has forbidden me,' he explained awkwardly.

'So you don't really like me then,' she suggested, winding him up.

'Yes. I do. I really do. But…'

'I'm going. If you can't help me. That's it. Goodbye,' she said, flouncing off.

Eddy was taken aback by this sudden change in their apparent relationship and stood gazing at her open mouthed as she walked away.

'Please don't go,' Eddy implored.

'I'm sorry Eddy, I helped you when you needed help. Have you forgotten?" she said, playing the guilt card. 'Now I'm asking for a small favour, that's all.'

'No, but...'

'Well, if you can't help me, then it's a bad deal,' she said, dramatically and flounced off again.

Eddy followed almost running to keep up.

'No, I want to help you but...'

'If you can't talk about the Institute, tell me what you know about this Doctor John then,' she demanded.

Eddy thought for a moment, the Doctor said not to talk about the hospital. He didn't say anything about not talking about himself.

'Oh, OK then,' Eddy agreed.

She smiled at his vulnerability.

'He drives a new car and he's got a new apartment,' Eddy revealed.

'So he's not living in the hospital anymore?' she queried.

'No. I think he has an apartment on the East Esplanade,' Eddy revealed.

'Does he have a girl friend?'

'I think he is very friendly with Laura from the hospital,' Eddy explained.

'That's interesting,' she thought.

'Umm...I heard her making a booking for a restaurant,' Eddy continued, conspiratorially.

'A restaurant booking! Really. Where?'

'I think it was the Surfers. I haven't been there myself, have you?'

'No, but I might have to introduce myself to them,' she thought. 'You didn't happen to overhear when?' she probed.

'I think it was Wednesday.'

'Wednesday! That's today,' she recalled. 'Ok Eddy, that's very good and helpful.'

'Are we friends again?' he asked desperately.

'Yes. Now you have given me that. But you mustn't say anything to Doctor John or Laura. I would like to surprise them there.'

'Oh that would be nice.' Eddy beamed, happy in the knowledge that they were friends again.

'I think we'll forget the café; I've just remembered something that I need to do,' Sophie said suddenly.

'Oh. OK,' Eddy said, disappointed that his date was being curtailed.

'Goodbye Eddy. Love you,' she said, giving him a peck on the cheek. But her mind was elsewhere, Sophie was already thinking of her next move to ingratiate herself to John and Laura.

Eddy stood and watched her go. 'She said she loved me, ' he said dreamily, touching his cheek.

'Right Doctor John. So you think that you can censor me do you? Well game on! There's many ways to skin a cat.' Sophie fumed. And started planning her retribution.

Chapter Fifty-six

Sophie's plan to interview John involved introducing herself casually and hope that her celebrity status would impress him. She hoped that while he was in a relaxed environment, he would grant her a subsequent interview.

Hence capitalising on the information that Eddy got for her about the dinner date with Laura, she booked herself in at the same restaurant.

She had called the restaurant and confirmed that they were indeed booked in. And, by claiming to be a friend who had forgotten when they were meeting, she found out the time too.

She had gone to town on her elegance, wearing a long black strapless evening gown, she was bejewelled with gold and pearl drop earrings. Around her long neck she wore a gold chain necklace with an icon of a TV award that she'd won, seductively disappearing into her cleavage. Around her wrist she wore a gold bangle and sported a pair of diamond encrusted rings on both hands.

She went to the beachside restaurant ahead of Laura and John's scheduled arrival time. By arriving early, she felt that she owned the space. Metaphorically, they would be coming into her territory.

She sat quietly waiting for their arrival, consuming several glasses of wine.

At last the pair arrived hand in hand, she heard the head waiter greet Laura by name.

Sophie recognised Laura from seeing her whilst protesting as Sheila, on the steps of the institute, with the anti-psychiatry mob. She had not seen John before but thought he looked very handsome in his smart cream jacket and grey slacks with the casual look of an open neck shirt.

Laura was wearing a light colourful summer dress with a revealing neckline, emphasizing her femininity and slim figure.

After they had been shown to their table, John chose to go to the bar to see the variety of available drinks, rather than giving the waiter an order.

Spotting him at the bar, Sophie casually sauntered over to him whilst he was ordering their drinks.

John was alerted to her approach by the heavy bouquet of her perfume, which preceded her.

'G'day,' she said. 'Do I know you? Your face is familiar,' Sophie asked.

'No I don't think so.' John said, studying her face and thinking he was being chatted up by a sex worker. But seeing her finery, he changed his assessment.

'You work at the hospital don't you?' she asked, confirming that she had the right person.

'Yes. Have I seen you there?' he wondered, checking his memory.

'No, but you might have seen me on the television,' she crowed. 'I've done a few documentaries,' she added modestly.

Immediately, alarm bells started ringing in his head. Was she that investigative reporter that the Professor had warned him about?

'Sorry, I very rarely watch television. So your fame is lost on me,' he informed her.

'Ohhh!' she blustered; her ego immediately deflated by his put down. People's usual reaction was to be overwhelmed by meeting a 'celebrity'.

I've heard so many good things about the hospital,' she lied. 'I wonder if I could interview you so you could explain about your work there?'

'No, sorry. Much too busy,' he lied.

Desperately she sought another approach.

'Is that a Canadian accent that I detect?' she asked.

'No, I'm English,' he explained, not wishing to go into the West country explanation. 'You'll excuse me, I must get back to my friend,' John said, picking up his drinks and going back to Laura, leaving Sophie stunned.

'Do you know who you were talking to at the bar?' Laura whispered, as he got back to their table.

'No. But she claimed to be something on TV,' he relayed, indifferently.

'Yes. She's that Investigative reporter, Sophie Mcbid, who exposes scandals. She's the one who rang the other day wanting an interview with the Professor.'

'Oh yes, I had my suspicions. She claimed to have seen me at the hospital,' John informed her. '

'Perhaps she's investigating you?' Laura joked, laughing.

'She might have heard about my motor racing reputation,' he suggested. 'Or that I'm a good lover,' he smiled, stroking Laura's thigh.

'So long as she isn't going to demand a performance test to check your reputation,' Laura smiled, putting her hand on his thigh, and squeezing it.

However, undaunted by John's lack of knowledge of her notoriety, Sophie wandered over to them.

'Sorry to disturb you. Do you mind if I join you?' she asked, putting her drink on their table, pre-empting an invitation.

'Well actually we…' John was going to say, yes he did mind. But Laura beat him to it.

'No, not at all,' Laura said politely. 'Bring a chair over.'

John flashed a look at his date. Sophie missed the glare as she struggled to drag a heavy chair over.

Laura looked at John, 'Don't struggle with that. John will help you. Won't you John?' she offered.

His look of disdain needed no words. Reluctantly he stood and moved to where Sophie was struggling with the chair. As he went to help her, their hands briefly touched on the arm of the chair. Enjoying the contact, she flashed him a smile but after a few seconds when he realised there was contact he quickly withdrew his hand.

'It's all yours,' she said, moving out of the way.'

John put the chair down next to his and sat down.

'It's so nice to see some friendly faces,' Sophie said, sitting and crossing her long legs.

'I do love your programmes,' Laura said, ingratiating herself.

'Oh that's very kind,' Sophie said, unconsciously patting her hair.

'Do you get a lot of grief from the people that you expose?' Laura continued.

'Yes, but it's all part of the territory,' the TV presenter said nonchalantly. 'You get a lot of nutters in all walks of life, don't you.'

John cleared his throat to suggest he disapproved of her terminology.

'Oh sorry Doctor. It is Doctor isn't it? I expect nutters is a term that you don't like hearing, as you work with mentally ill people.'

'Doctor is right, although I am actually a qualified psychiatrist. Yes I've had medical training. But primarily I am an expert in mental health.' John said stiffly, not really wanting to discuss his job. 'And, yes, you're right. I don't like that disparaging term.'

'Please accept my apologies for my inappropriate language,' Sophie said, cursing herself for her alcoholically fuelled gaff. 'Not the best way to get him on her side,' she thought.

'People with mental health issues have genuine problems that require professional assistance. We use all the tools at our disposal to help them live a 'normal life'; John continued. 'Although I dislike that term, too. It depends on what you define as 'normal.'

'Oh yes it's a bit of a 'minefield' isn't it?' Sophie said, condescendingly.

'Now if you don't mind let's change the subject,' John suggested.

'Yes of course. I appreciate that you're off duty...but I had heard of some strange goings on in the hospital,' Sophie continued.

'I'm sorry, Miss. Whatever your name is. I am having a quiet drink here; I am not doing an interview,' John said haughtily.

'Apologies. Force of habit. Umm perhaps I could interview you at a more convenient time?' she said, cursing herself for her impatience to get him talking.

'Yes, but I'm very busy and I've not got my diary with me. Look, give me your card and I'll call you. Now if you wouldn't mind, Laura and I are having a quiet drink,' the psychiatrist said coldly.

Sophie dug into her handbag and pulled out a business card.

'Well, I'll look forward to speaking to you soon,' she said, offended by John's dismissal, 'And goodbye to you. It was nice meeting you Laura.'

'You too,' Laura replied demurely.

'Yes, goodbye,' John said dismissively.

As Sophie stormed off, clearly annoyed, Laura said, 'You were very rude to her John. I hope any subsequent report she makes doesn't present you in a bad light. These TV people can bend the truth you know. Especially if they don't like you,' Laura counselled, quietly.

'I'm not worried. I can hold my own,' he said nonchalantly. 'Now where were we,' he said putting his hand back on her thigh.

Following their lovely meal and a few drinks they retired back to John's apartment. And resumed their intimacy.

After many moments of passion, in the early hours, Laura slowly unpeeled herself from him.

'Aren't you going to stay all night? he asked cuddling her.

'I'd love to, but I've got an early start tomorrow,' she revealed. 'The Professor wants me to cover a breakfast meeting with him. I need some sleep rather than your body.'

'Well if you have to go, I'll see you off the premises,' he said, getting out of bed and nuzzling her neck while she dressed.

John put on his dressing gown and went down in the lift with her.

She unlocked her car and they kissed before she climbed in. 'Missing you already,' he said breathlessly.

Having made sure that she was safely in her car, John watched her drive off and returned to bed and was quickly asleep. Unaware that their passionate goodbye had been observed.

Chapter Fifty-seven

'Ding dong.'

John stirred sluggishly and peered at his watch. His eyes slowly focussed.

'Three o'clock in the morning. Who the hell is ringing my door bell at this time of day?' he muttered. 'Oh god has Laura had a problem?' he panicked.

'Ding Dong,' the door bell sounded again. He dragged himself out of bed and quickly made his way to the door monitor screen, half asleep.

He remotely switched on the porch light and stared at the face on the monitor. It wasn't Laura after all, but Sophie was stood there, leaning against the porch support.

'Oh it's you,' John muttered. 'What the hell are you doing at my door at this time of the morning?'

'My car has broken down,' she explained.'

'Well I'm not a garage mechanic,' he said irritably.

'I know but I need help.'

'Anyway, what are you doing driving at this time of night?' he said annoyed.

'Work,' she informed him. 'Can I come in and ring my garage?'

'What's wrong with using a phone box?' he asked suspiciously.

'They are all out of order, I'm afraid,' she lied, having not even tried any.

Still sleep fogged, he flicked the door lock switch and allowed her in. 'You'll have to use the lift, I'm on the top floor,' he informed her.

Clad only in his pyjama trousers, he opened the door to his apartment and listened to the lift humming up to his floor.

The lift door opened and she made her way towards him.

After leaving the restaurant because of John's rudeness, Sophie had gone home with her tail between her legs but reluctant to let go of a possible interview, she hatched a plot to get back at him.

She had changed from her evening wear and removed all her jewellery. Instead she was wearing a short plain dress with a low cut neckline and showing a fair amount of cleavage. Her heady perfume filled the hall as she entered.

'My, what a fine figure of a man,' she said, studying his bare muscled torso. I've been walking for an hour trying to find a working phone box,' she lied. 'And I'm parched. You don't think I could have a coffee please,' she asked.

In reality, she had been staking out John's apartment, having already spotted Laura's distinctive car parked near-by. So anticipating that Laura would leave at some time she waited to get John alone.

It had been a long vigil and at one stage she was going to give up, deciding that Laura was staying the night, but her patience had finally paid off.

She waited for another half hour after Laura had left and the lights had gone out in the apartment and then rang the doorbell.

'You've got a nerve,' he said leading her into the lounge. 'There's the phone,' he pointed. 'Against my better judgement I'll make you a coffee. I'm not a bleeding café you know,' he muttered disgruntled, pulling on his dressing gown.

As he left her, she retrieved a small spy camera out of her handbag and started photographing the room, keeping an ear out for his return.

After finishing the filming she wandered over to the phone and wrote his telephone number down. She took the receiver off, at the same time scanning the room for anything else that would prove useful. Then she spotted his briefcase stored between two lounge chairs.

Satisfied that he was still in the kitchen preparing her coffee, she picked the briefcase up and slid the catches on it, and to her delight found that it was not locked.

She quickly opened it and found several files inside, one of which interested her. Labelled 'Eddy Jones'.

She scan read a few pages and found an entry for his drug regime. The name Phenloramide caught her eye. It was the same drug that Eddy had reported that had been used for the three dead patients and had been mentioned at the recent inquests. She quickly photographed several pages.

His coffee preparations finished; she could hear John walking back towards the lounge. Taken by surprise, she didn't have time to put the file back, so hid it behind her back as he entered.

Spotting the phone off the hook, he asked 'did you contact the garage?'

'It was just ringing out with no reply and I got bored holding it so I put it down,' she lied. 'I'll have to get a taxi and sort the car out in the morning. Of course, if you were a gentleman you'd offer to take me home yourself,' she purred.

'Well you obviously don't know me well enough, I'm definitely not a gentleman. And a taxi ride will allow me to go to bed. Here, drink your coffee while I find the taxi number.'

He left the room again, so she hastily stuffed the file back in the briefcase, just in time as he returned..

'The coffee is delicious thank you,' she said picking her cup up. 'Were you not going to have one?'

'As soon as I get rid of you, I'm back to bed. Here's the taxi number,' he said proffering her a business card.

'Thank you,' she said, putting down her cup and taking the card. She moved to the phone and rang the number. After a few minutes, he could hear the despatcher answer.

'G'day, I would like a taxi please to collect me from,' and gave John's address. John later wondered how she knew his address without him telling her.

'We'll be there in fifteen minutes,' the despatcher said.

'Thank you,' she said and hung up.

Chapter Fifty-eight

'So what are you doing out at this time of the night?' John demanded. 'Sensible people are normally in bed.'

'Us investigators tend to roam around looking for stories at any time night or day,' she replied. 'I'm dying for a wee, may I use your toilet?'

'If you must,' he uttered, reluctantly. 'It's along the corridor second on the right.'

'Thank you,' she said grabbing her handbag and following his directions.

After using the toilet, she crept back along the corridor looking in several rooms until she found and entered the master bedroom. The bed was obviously unmade as a result of her disturbing his sleep.

Ensuring he was still in the lounge she took several photographs of his bed and bedroom.

She couldn't have anticipated that this great opportunity would present itself to compromise him somehow. Quickly she reviewed her options. From 'managed' situations accumulated throughout her journalistic career, she had developed various 'dirty tricks' to undermine her victims credibility.

If she could get John in a compromising situation, perhaps she could blackmail him into helping her with her investigations. And being here, in his bedroom, was the perfect opportunity.

She wandered around the room touching things, pulling out some hair and putting it in his bed and under his pillow. All the while sowing her forensic signature to prove she had been in there.

As she wandered around his bedroom she became more focussed on wanting to do something more to compromise him. Should she leave a pair of her knickers under the bed to imply that he'd had sex with her. No, she discounted that. He'd probably find them and be alerted.

'Now how can I set this guy up to make sure that he cooperates with me?' she wondered. 'Ah! What have we here?' she said to herself, spotting several used condoms on the carpet.

'It looks like they had a few intimate moments earlier. Although, I don't think much of his personal hygiene, leaving used condoms around is a bit unsavoury,' she thought. 'In my possession, however, perhaps one could come in handy.'

Ensuring it was tied, to prevent leakage, she put a used durex in her handbag.

'I think they can match blood type from semen,' she thought. 'With the condom I can manufacture the evidence to take to the Police if he won't cooperate. I'm sure that I could convince him, if necessary, that with some on my knickers, bra, or dress that I could say that he had raped me.

But hopefully he will comply with my investigations and it won't get that far,' she beamed at her cunning plan.

Her self-congratulations was short lived as she heard him coming along the corridor.

Realising that she wasn't still in the toilet, and checking the other rooms, he burst in to his bedroom. 'What the hell are you doing in here?' he ranted angrily.

'I was just admiring it, that's all. It really is very lovely. Just like the rest of your apartment,' Sophie gushed.

'Well get the hell out you nosey bitch,' he ordered angrily. 'Thank god your taxi has just arrived,' he said, seeing the lights of the cab pulling up outside.

'Thank you for your 'hospitality'' she uttered sarcastically, leaving his bedroom, and going ahead of him. 'Sorry to have disturbed your sleep.'

'Good night,' he said opening the apartment door.

Irritated by the nosey woman, John slammed the door behind her and listened to the lift going down and the outside door being closed.

Had he watched the taxi leave, he would have seen the cab just pull up next to her car around the corner.

As she drove off she thought. 'I now have a means to an end. You'll be sorry for refusing to talk to me,' she smiled to herself evilly.

Chapter Fifty-nine

Sophie rang John's home telephone, several days after her intrusive late night visit to his apartment. She had obtained the number, surreptitiously when calling the garage to 'so say' rescue her.

'John Masters, whose calling?'

'G'day John, it's Sophie.'

'Sophie?' he queried. 'Sophie who?'

'The Sophie who you kindly helped out when my car broke down.'

'Oh. It's you, is it?' he said stiffly.

'I just rang to say thanks and apologise for waking you up in the middle of the night.'

'Yes well don't make a habit of it. I won't be so obliging next time. Goodbye,' he said aiming to hang up.

'Umm, just before you hang up, I figured that as you hadn't got around to ringing me. I thought I'd save you the bother in order to arrange the interview date,' she said.

'You needn't have bothered. I wasn't going to ring you anyway,' he said tersely.

'Oh, that's a pity because I was hoping that you could help me with my investigations.'

'Investigations! What investigations?' Already aware that something was a foot, John played dumb.

'Investigations into the failings of the Mental Health system, that I'm planning to cover in a documentary.'

'What gives you the impression that it's a failing system?'

'Well several indicators that have been flagged up to me. But I thought you'd be the right informed person to consult to help me identify fact from fiction.'

'Really and why do you think that?'

'There have been several deaths of patients from your hospital and I believe at least one autopsy showed signs of some significant brain damage. I wonder if you'd like to comment.'

'No I wouldn't. Patient confidentiality and hospital procedures prevent me from commenting on anything formally.'

'What about informally?'

'No. You need to talk to the Professor about that,' John informed her firmly.

'Only your patient, Eddy, I believe, has been telling me stuff about you and the Professor.'

'Well anything that Eddy says must be treated with a pinch of salt, due to his health issues,' the psychiatrist suggested.

'Something about, arguing over the merits of the trial drugs and the conflict with your new hypnotherapy treatment,' she lied, making an informed guess.

'Yes Eddy is a patient. But he is in no position to know about any hospital procedures. He has given you erroneous information. You need to speak to the Professor,' John repeated irritably.

'What tale has Eddy spun her I wonder.' John thought. 'Clearly my subliminal instructions not to tell Sheila anything didn't work.'

'Oh that's a pity because I've a problem and I'm hesitating about whether to go to the police or not, Sophie explained.'

'What's that to do with me?'

'Everything, because you raped me.'

'What? When I did what?' John said in amazement. 'What the hell are you talking about. Raping you? Are you mad?'

'No I'm not mad. Don't you remember? When I came to seek help because my car had broken down. You took advantage of me and raped me in your bedroom.'

'You are deluded. I never touched you.'

'Yes you did.'

'Where has this come from? You know that's not true.'

'Yes I know that, but the police don't. And as a victim of a serious sexual assault, they will believe me. Especially when they find your blood type in the semen on my clothes.'

'Semen! I've never been anywhere near you. Let alone had any sexual activity with you,' John argued vehemently

'No, but your shoddy housekeeping leaving used condoms on the bedroom floor after your session with Laura, I assume. Will help me prove my case.'

'So that's what you were doing in my bedroom. You nosey scheming bitch.'

'No need to get like that,' she soothed. 'I'm sure we can work something out and keep things civilised.'

'I wondered what had happened to that condom. In the end I convinced myself that I had flushed it away,' he said.'

'Yes and now I have it and I think I have you too,' she crowed. 'You help me and I'll destroy it and my stained underclothes. If you don't help me, I'll accuse you of rape. My accusation alone will ruin you and your reputation. You know what happens, as soon as I publicly accuse you, you WILL become a rapist in most people's eyes. Innocent or not. Mud sticks. The damage will be done,' she concluded, pleased with her evil scheme.

'You conniving bitch,' he spat angrily.

'I've found whilst doing this job, that often the end justifies the means in uncovering scandalous activities. Especially if I can get celebrity out of it,' she thought.

'So what's it to be?' she demanded.

For the first time in his life, John was lost for words.

Chapter Sixty

Eventually, Sophie persuaded John to meet her in a deserted beachside car park.

'Sorry about this clandestine cloak and dagger stuff,' she said, getting in to his car. 'But I find it's best to minimise visibility during these investigations, it stops nosey newspaper journalists leaking possible leads.'

'I really don't know why I've agreed to meet you,' John told her angrily. 'Your vile lies can be scientifically overturned,' he bluffed.

'Do you want to take the chance that they will? Even if they are, after my accusations, the damage will be done to your reputation,' she reminded him.

'Just remember your lies will be found out and your reputation will go out the window too,' he warned her.

'Don't worry, I've done this before. I know the score and the way out,' she boasted. 'Now, I know that the Professor is up to no good and I am determined to expose the scandal.'

'To my knowledge, you are barking up the wrong tree. The Professor is merely conducting advanced scientific research which will hopefully be of great benefit to those suffering from mental illness,' John said sincerely.

'Your loyalty to the Professor is misplaced,' she derided. 'Make sure that when I sink his ship that you're not on board.'

'Why do you want to damage the man's reputation? He is the recognised expert in the field. He is trying to help millions worldwide who suffer from various forms of mental illness.'

'Yes, but his methods are questionable, using his patients as guinea pigs to bolster his own inflated ego. I know for a fact that at least three have died on his trial. And I believe there are many more who are likely to, as well,' she suggested.

'There is no proof that their death is directly linked to the trial,' John said firmly. 'Indeed one was murdered.'

'No, but the neuropathologist that examined the unfortunate Digger Lucas's brain can. He found traces of your Professors drugs in the eaten away section of the losers brain.'

'It proves nothing. All medication circulates throughout the blood stream,' John explained. 'I believe the cause of death was a stab wound anyway.'

'Yes but his death exposed something that the Professor has been hiding. His drug trial is nothing worse than a scandal, similar to Doctor Mengele during the second world war.'

'Never. You can't possibly compare that Nazi murderer to the Professor's ground breaking work.' he said, forcefully refuting her explanation.

'If you don't believe me, take a look at the cause of death on these death certificates that I managed to get my hands on,' she said showing John a handful of forged documents.

'Death certificates? he queried, taking the forged documents from her.

'Yes, quite revealing, aren't they?'

'How did you get hold of these?' John demanded, thumbing through the pile. 'There must be at least twenty here,' he pointed out.

'I have got my ways. It's a means to an end. All of these were secretly on the Professors drug trial. Fishy isn't it?'

In reality during her meticulous preparations for the forthcoming documentary, Sophie had commissioned a graphic designer from the Television company to draw up false death certificates. The documents made it look as if many more people had died as a result of the Professors drug trial.

As his skills were normally used for creating imagery of feasible documentation for various television productions, the designer thought nothing of Sophie's request.

'I don't know. I'm sure that there is a logical reason for it,' John said, taken aback.

'I think it is proof that your Professor is clearly hiding something. These people are nothing other than 'crash test dummies' to be injected with nefarious drugs.'

'All speculation,' John said defensively.

'They were probably 'John Dos' with no relatives so that nobody cares whether they live or die.'

'What proof have you got?'

'I think these death certificates are a good start, don't you?

'Not necessarily.'

I think he could be 'in bed' with the pharmaceutical company to line his own pockets,' she accused. 'His work has nothing to do with creating a world beating drug to tackle mental illness. It's all about making and selling a fake drug which has as much healing power as an aspirin,' she fictionalised. He is probably manipulating the results even as we speak.'

'Against a dedicated and well respected scientist like the Professor, why should I believe someone like you? You clearly have the morals of the gutter,' John said angrily.

'Steady now. You are in danger of pissing me off and I might not be so understanding about the circumstances of your sexual attack on me.'

'You're despicable,' he fumed.

'Comes with the job, I'm afraid. It's what happens when I constantly have to deal with lowlife people. Some of it rubs off. So long as I expose the scandals, then I'm happy,' she explained.

'I'll think about it,' John said, thrusting the death certificates back at her.

'I've a list of specific bits of information that I want from you,' she said taking another document from her file.

'Have you? Well, you'll have to wait until I've decided what I'm going to do then aren't you?'

'I warn you that it's not an idle threat. If you don't play ball, I'll present all the alleged rape evidence to the police.'

'And then you won't get anything from me,' he called her bluff.

'I've other sources that I can tap,' she replied, double bluffing.

'As I said I'll think about it.'

'Don't think about it too long because there might be a new scandal that I've unearthed. Involving patients who have been drugged and sexually assaulted as well.'

White hot with anger, John ordered her out of his car and before she'd barely slammed the passenger door, he raced out of the car park in a cloud of tyre smoke, leaving a grinning Sophie.

'Coming together nicely,' she thought.

Chapter Sixty-one

John couldn't settle. He drove to the beach and wandered up and down the shore line, hoping that an idea would come to him. Getting rid of the threat would be the ideal, but killing Sophie was not going to be his solution.

Desperately trying to find an acceptable resolution, he finally decided to tell Laura about Sophie's threats and hoped by sharing his problem that he would find a way forward.

Finally he telephoned her from a public kiosk.

'Imagine institute. How may I help?'

'Laura, it's me, John.'

'Hello stranger, I was wondering where you were.'

'I've got something on my mind. I need to talk to you about.'

'OK, no problem,' she said, concerned.

'Come round to my place after you've finished this afternoon.'

'Yes OK. Are you sure that you're alright?'

'Yes. I'll see you later.'

'OK.'

John heard her arrive at the apartment and opened the door before she could put her key in the lock. He gave her a big hug.

'Are you sure that you are alright John?' she queried suspiciously, returning the hug.

'Yes, well no,' he said, closing the door behind her.

'What's all the mystery about?' Laura asked putting her handbag down and getting two glasses of iced water for them from the refrigerator.

'I've got a problem with that nosey reporter. You know the one that forced herself on us at the restaurant the other day?'

'Yes, Sophie Mcbid. See, I told you to be kind to her. You walked into a vipers nest there. What sort of problem? Is she stalking you?' Laura joked.

'No. It's worse than that....She's blackmailing me,' he revealed.

'Blackmail! What do you mean blackmail? What have you done for her to blackmail you?' Laura demanded suspiciously.

'That's just it. I haven't done anything. She is...is contriving a fictional story to say that I raped her.'

'You what?' Laura said in astonishment.

'She is saying that I raped her,' John repeated, uncomfortably.

'And did you?' Laura quizzed.

'No of course not.' John refuted irritably.

'Well then you've got nothing to worry about then have you? I mean the whole thing is clearly a pack of lies, isn't it?' she asked, studying his face, seeking reassurance.

'Yes it is,' he confirmed.

'Well you've got nothing to worry about then, have you?' she repeated.

'Well it's not that straightforward,' John explained awkwardly.

'What do you mean? Not straight forward? Did you drag her off the street? '

'No.'

'Take advantage of her on the beach? What?' Laura demanded, frantically.

'None of those things. Of course not.' John denied emphatically. 'The thing is, after you left the other night, she came here, at three o'clock in the morning, claiming that her car had broken down.'

'You didn't tell me about that,' Laura said sceptically.

'No. I didn't. I didn't think it was important,' John said, now beginning to realise that he had made a mistake by not telling Laura before.

'A woman coming to your door at three o'clock in the morning, not important!' Laura said suspiciously.

'I...I didn't think anything of it. She came and was gone within fifteen minutes.'

'Oh John!' Laura said, nervously putting her hands to her mouth.

'I let her in to use my phone. I gave her a cup of coffee and she used the toilet. She was a long time coming back after using the toilet and I found her in my bedroom.'

'So what did you do?' she asked apprehensively.

'I asked her, what the hell she was doing in there and I told her to clear off.'

'And did she?'

'Yes.'

'So nothing happened then?' she queried.

'No, no of course not,' John said emphatically.

'So why are you worried ? How do you know about this rape allegation?'

'A few days later she rang me. And told me she wanted to do the interview with me about the Institute. I told her no.'

'What did she say?'

'She wanted me to provide her with personal information about the Professor and his trial.'

'What did you say?'

'I told her there would be no interview and to speak to the Professor herself.'

'What did she say?'

'That she would tell the police that I'd raped her.'

'So out of the blue, with no evidence, she's going to say that you raped her?' she said incredulously.

'Yes.'

'Well, if you didn't touch her, you don't have anything to worry about surely?'

'Unfortunately, she took a condom that we used when you were here earlier.'

'A what?'

'A condom.'

'Is she perverted or what? What the hell is she going to do with that?'

'Sprinkle my semen from the condom on her underwear as proof that I had sex with her,' John explained.

'The sick bitch. How will that prove it was you?' she demanded.

'The forensic people will probably be able to match my blood type,' he explained.

'Oh my god. John, that is…that is awful. I'm lost for words. The conniving bitch.'

'I feel exactly the same.'

'So what does she want from you? Money?' Laura asked.

'No. She wants information about the Professor and his trial,' John amplified.

'The Professor and his trial? Why?'

'She is doing a programme on him and his, according to her, his scandalous activities with a pharmaceutical company, whilst using patients as guinea pigs.

'Yeah but all trials are like that. I can assure you that it's properly reported,' Laura divulged. 'I know, I type up the reports.'

'Yes but there's more. Is the trial approved? The Professor suggested that it wasn't.'

'Oh heavens! If that's the case he could be in a lot of trouble,' Laura revealed.'

'She is also suggesting that he is taking backhanders from the pharmaceutical company to slew the trial results. But that could be lies too. She even showed me several death certificates from people who 'so say' were on the trial that have died and they have not been listed in the official trial figures.'

'How did she get those?' Death certificates are not issued freely.' Laura pointed out.

'I don't know. She reckons she has a lot of contacts that are on her wavelength in exposing wrongdoing.'

'This is awful.'

'But the Professors alleged misdeeds isn't helping me,' John grumbled.

'Well surely you've got no option have you? You've got to go to the Police and tell them she is framing you for something you haven't done in order to blackmail you?'

'If I do that then I'll potentially incriminate myself by telling them of the rape allegation. I'm frightened that they will believe her. She's a very forceful character. And it's conceivable that the police will agree with the old adage, 'there's no smoke without fire' and charge me anyway.'

'Well, blackmail is a serious crime too. You must go to the Police and tell them about her threats,' Laura insisted.

'If I do that, it will arouse their suspicions. Then how do I clear my name? They will probably have to arrest me. No, best to keep the law out of it,' he argued.

'Then you've got to tell her what she wants to know, otherwise she will ruin your career. All those years of studying will have been for nothing,' Laura countered.

'I fear that if I give in to her blackmail this time, that will only be the start of it. She will want more and more information and I'll end up undermining my ethical standards.'

'What sort of information is she after anyway?' Laura queried.

'I'm not sure but I would imagine something about trial statistics, volume of people successfully treated. Numbers who have died. The cost: the Professors aim; Is the Professor being paid by a Pharmaceutical company to develop the drug? What's the name of the company? the link between Prof and Pharm company? etc ' John said.

'Well that's not earth shattering though is it?' Laura observed. 'I mean if it will remove the rape threat...'

'But if I bow to her demands, it's like admitting that I'm guilty.'

'And are you?' Laura repeated.

'No of course not.' he reiterated angrily. 'I need a few days to think about it.'

'Oh, John. What a horrible situation.'

'Surely, there must be another way. I just need to find it,' John said desperately.

Chapter Sixty-two

Eddy arrived at Johns office at the appointed time for his next hypnotherapy treatment.

'Come in and take a seat, Eddy,' the psychiatrist invited, indicating a chair near him.

'Thank you.'

'Before we start today. Can you tell me, how long has the Professor been prescribing tablets for you?'

'Always...a...a long time. I don't know how long though,' Eddy replied.

'When did it actually start, can you remember?'

'Ever since I've been here. Sometimes it's different colour tablets that the Professor gives me.'

'Ok, not to worry. I'll speak to the Professor about it myself.'

'Why do you want to know?' Eddy asked.

'I want to assess what we would need to do, if we took you off those tablets,' John informed his patient.

''Are you going to take me off the trial then?' Eddy queried.

'It's a possibility. But don't worry. I'll discuss it with the Professor first.'

'Are you going to hypnotise me again today Doctor?' Eddy asked, standing up and moving towards the couch.

'No, you can stay where you are. I have some good news.'

'Good news?'

'Yes, I think I've got to the bottom of your problems.'

'The bottom of my problems! Oh, that's good news. Isn't it?' he wondered.

'Yes it's very good, because it means we can start giving you the correct treatment for your problems,' John said enthusiastically.

'But does that mean we won't have our chats again? Because I like talking to you. It makes me feel special,' Eddy revealed.

'Well I too have enjoyed the investigation. I've enjoyed digging into your past to find out your issues,' John admitted.

'Oh, I'm so excited,' Eddy jiggled. 'My past. Wow!'

'I've discovered that your problems stem from a car accident that happened when you were a child.'

Eddy's smile faded.

'Since it happened all those many years ago you have bravely buried your emotions about the incident. However, by doing so, it has affected your mental health.'

'Oh! I never knew.'

'I think the cause of your problem has been that you have never grieved properly over the loss of your father. You have bottled it all up inside. Your emotions need to be allowed to come out.'

Oh I remember now!' Eddy screwed his face up as he dug into the recesses of his memory. After a few moments of inner thought Eddy looked up and stared at John, his eyes moist with tears. 'I loved my dad...He told me I had to be strong if I was ever going to be a doctor.

John was pleased to hear Eddy's recollection remembering vital facts. It was a major milestone. Eddy had overcome the fog in his mind caused by decades of drugs.

'Yes, that's right. Being a doctor does mean that you do have to learn to become detached from your patients grief. But, doctors are human beings too. They still need to grieve for their own losses,' the psychiatrist explained.

John's own grief, over the death of his girlfriend in the UK, was still raw.

Eddy, I know from personal experience how hard grief is to deal with. The black abys of grief never goes away. But the grieving gets easier as time passes.

Look at it this way. Imagine our loss is a black circle, a deep black hole. Surrounding that circle, that hole, is our grief. Immediately after our loss we hug the circle and constantly revisit it, distraught at our loss. As time passes our grieving moves away from frequently touching the blackness and we are able to cope better. But deep within, the sadness never goes away.

'I was strong. I never cried,' Eddy boasted.

'That's a pity, because, especially as a child, you needed to let your emotions out. I am sure if you had cried, your Dad would still have been proud of you anyway,' John suggested.

'Do you know, I go to talk to him at the cemetery every other day. He knows all about you.' Eddy divulged. 'You know sometimes I think you look like my dad if you didn't have that beard.' Eddy observed.

'Well I can't comment on that, I don't know what your dad looked like. However, what I'd like to do is to take you back to the forest where the accident occurred to finally help you address your bottled up emotions.'

'Go back? Oh no, no, I…I don't. No…I don't think that's a good idea. I don't want to go back there,' Eddy said standing, starting to become tearful. 'No…no.'

'Ok, no problem Eddy. I'm not going to force you. If you don't want to go back that is fine too. Sometimes it helps to confront what you fear by tackling it head on. What often happens is that your imagination conjures up scenarios which are more frightening than actually facing the real problem,' the psychiatrist explained gently.

'No. I don't want to. No thank you. Can I go now?' Eddy said nervously moving towards the door.

'Yes. Of course you can. But if you change your mind, let me know and we'll arrange something,' John informed him.

'Ok.'

Eddy ran home, fearful that John would catch up with him and force him to face his demons anyway.

When Eddy got to the sheltered housing, he barged straight into Marilyn's house, without knocking.

'Have you been with that woman again?' Marilyn demanded.

'No, I've been with Doctor John,' Eddy panted.

'Oh, the shrink?'

'Yes. He wants me to go back to where he thinks my problems started in a car crash. But I don't want to go,' Eddy confessed.

'Where is it?'

'I'm not sure. It's a long way away though, I think.'

'Well why don't you? It would be great to get away from this dump for a bit,' she suggested.

'Yeah, I suppose. But I'm scared,' Eddy revealed.

'What are you scared of,' she asked, puzzled.

'I…I don't know,' he confessed.

'If you like, I'll come with you and protect you,' she said, punching her fist into the palm of her open hand to reinforce her point.

'Umm, I'm not sure,' he said, hesitantly.

'Up to you,' she offered.

'Would you?' Eddy asked, apprehensively.

'Yes, of course. I haven't been away from this place for years,' she added.

'I'll have to ask Doctor John if that's Ok first,' Eddy informed her.

'Oh that would be brilliant if you could,' Marilyn said, giving him a bear hug.

Chapter Sixty-three

After giving Marilyn's offer some more thought, Eddy decided that he must be braver, like her and face his demons. So he returned to the Institute and tracked John down to his office.

'Back so soon Eddy?' the psychiatrist said, as Eddy entered.

'Yes…ummm…Doctor John I've been thinking, and if you still want me to go to that place you mentioned. I'll go…but only if Marilyn can come with me,' Eddy informed the Doctor.

'Marilyn too? Oh and why's that?'

'Because I'm scared. And she will protect me,' Eddy advised him.

'But there is nothing to be frightened of Eddy. I'll be with you,' John assured him.

'No. Unless Marilyn comes with me, I'm not going,' Eddy said firmly, crossing his arms across his chest, defiantly.

'That might be difficult to arrange then. I anticipate that the Professor will take some persuasion in letting you go in the first place, let alone taking someone else as well.'

'Then I won't go,' Eddy said firmly.

'There is another complication. If Marilyn comes, I'll have to get a female to chaperone her too,' John explained. 'I'm not sure that the Professor will agree to four of us going.'

Eddy was resolute in his terms. 'Marilyn or neither of us,' he stated finally.

'Ok, I'll give it a try. But I'm not promising anything, I'll let you know,' John informed him.

'Thank you,' Eddy said, not sure that he wanted to go anyway, in spite of Marilyn's promise to protect him.

John subsequently made his way to the Professor's office and entered at the others invitation.

'Yes John, what can I do for you? 'the Professor said looking up from his report.

'I would like to take Eddy off site to the Kosciuszko National Park to address the roadblock in his mind.'

'Off site! To a national park? This is most unusual. Why?

'I've discovered that his problems all stem back to a crash in which his father died, when he was a child.'

'In the Kosciuszko National Park?'

'Yes. He blames himself for his father's death and he has never grieved properly. I believe that by taking him back to the site of his trauma we might be able to exorcise his mental issues.'

'John, I think you have already spent far too much time on this exercise to address the root cause of Eddy's problems. I don't think there is sufficient medical evidence that will justify the cost.'

'On the contrary, trauma therapy is an emerging way of treating certain types of mental health issues and I believe Eddy would benefit from the exercise.'

'What can you possibly achieve by going to a location several decades after the event? What conceivable benefit will he gain from the trip?' the Professor demanded.

'It's all about releasing his fears. It's the trigger that is holding him back. The mental roadblock.'

'So you haven't been able to cure him yet then?' the Professor asked sceptically.

'Not yet no. 'It's a multistep process.'

'I told you that your hypnotherapy wouldn't work. And you think a holiday in the forest will?' the academic ridiculed John's suggestion.

'The hypnotherapy has revealed the cause of Eddy's brain block. This blockage is preventing him from being able to move on with his life,' John explained, ignoring the Professor's barbed observations.

'Even if I agree to let you take him away…'

'Them,' John interrupted.

'Them! What do you mean them? I thought we were talking about Eddy.'

'Yes, we are, but…'

'So are you now talking about taking a coach load on the trip?'

'No, just Marilyn…'

'Why Marilyn?'

'Well you know, those two are joined at the hip. Eddy is scared to go without his bodyguard. And of course if Marilyn comes, then I'd need to take a woman chaperone and was thinking of asking Laura.'

'God, you don't want much do you? Well, sorry there's no money in the budget anyway for this type of therapy,' the Professor said dismissively.

'Ok, no problem. I'll fund it from my research grant,' John countered. 'It's not going to cost that much. It's only about a 500 kilometres road trip.

'So if you go, how long is this 'beano' going to take?'

'Well because of the distance, I plan just one overnight stop,' John advised.

'So now you are talking about not only the trip but overnight accommodation and meals as well?'

'Yes.'

'Well I hope your grant is sufficient to cover it,' the Professor pointed out.

'If it will sort Eddy out permanently, I think it is a good use of my grant,' John rationalised.

'Well against my better judgement, I'll agree. BUT only if you ensure that they continue to take their medication while they're away. They must continue to be part of my trial,' the Professor insisted.

'Talking about trials, that reminds me. I couldn't find any records in Eddy's file about his current medication,' John revealed. 'So I added my own notes about the drugs you have put him on during this trial.'

'No well, I…I err. Took it out to update it. That'll be why. It shouldn't have any impact on your trip anyway.'

'No, perhaps not,' John agreed.

'Anyway. I suppose there is a silver lining to your trip.'

'Which is?'

'Hopefully with Marilyn off the scene, the confrontations and violent incidents around here will cease,' the academic suggested. 'At least for a short time anyway.'

'Thank you. I've every confidence that Eddy will benefit from the experience,' John said.

'I don't share your optimism,' the Professor added as John left.

Chapter Sixty-four

John went straight to Laura and explained his proposal.

'So you're asking me to spend several days in close contact with two patients?'

'Yes, that's just about it. But at least you'll be away from the office phone and all those complaints from the neighbours,' John reasoned.

'I suppose there is that,' she said, warming to the idea.

'And they have to stay on their medication too,' John added.

'Ok. So what's the itinerary?'

'We're going near to the town of Jindabyne in the Kosciuszko national park, where Eddy revealed under hypnosis, the location of the accident site. Can you dig out any information about it please?' John asked.

'Such as what?'

'I don't know, anything you can find. Actual location of the accident site would be good.'

'Yes I suppose the local newspaper archives ought to have some details. Leave it with me,' Laura confirmed.

'I suggest we travel down on the first day, stay overnight, visit the crash site on the following day and journey home later that day. So we will need some accommodation nearby,' John added.

'What about a car?' she probed.

'I'm quite happy to take mine. It will be good to give the 'Beamer' a long run. It's just the four of us and overnight luggage anyway,' John confirmed.

'What about the cost? Has the Professor authorised it?'

'No he didn't to start off with. But I eventually persuaded him and I'm funding it from my research grant, so it doesn't impact on the Institutes finances,' John informed her.

'So what date did you have in mind?'

'Sooner rather than later. You have access to my diary, so take your pick. I've nothing pressing at the moment.'

'Ok.'

'As soon as possible. I don't want Eddy to talk himself out of it or for Marilyn to get locked up because she's been brawling again.'

'I thought this was all about Eddy? Why is Marilyn coming?'

'Eddy won't go without her,' John explained.

'So it's accommodation for four of us, is that right?' Laura checked.

'Yes.'

'Ok leave it with me,' Laura confirmed.

John went to see Eddy in his house.

'Good news Eddy, the Professor has agreed that we can take you to the park, where it all happened.'

'Oh really?' Eddy said, now not so sure. 'What about Marilyn is she coming too?'

'Yes and Laura will be Marilyn's chaperone,' John informed him.

'Oh…that's good then,' Eddy replied nervously. 'And Marilyn can come as well, you promise?'

'Yes Marilyn can come to keep you company,' John repeated.

Chapter Sixty-five

Laura got the Kosciuszko national park to dig into their newspaper archives to find an article about the accident.

Eventually after a painstaking search, including trawling through the fire service log book archives, they were able to find the newspaper article that referred to the crash.

When the archivist rang to tell her of their success Laura was over the moon.

'Would you be able to fax a copy to me?' Laura asked.

'Sure, give me your fax number.'

Laura gave her the number, checked that her machine had sufficient thermal paper on the roll for the incoming message and waited with bated breath for the fax machine number to ring.

Finally it rang and she heard the fax machines do their electronic handshake before the distant fax transmitted the data.

Laura watched and listened with mounting excitement to the strange tones as the black and white image revealed itself on her fax machine.

Finally the call finished, she ripped the thermal paper off the machine and gave it a cursory glance and then rushed up stairs to John's office, bursting into the room in excitement.

'Here you are John. Here's the information that I've been digging for,' she puffed. 'Eddy's incident was well reported. This is the article,' she said giving him the fax copy.

'Thank you,' he said with mounting excitement.

'It's a brief article and a not very good image of a photograph,' Laura explained. 'It hasn't scanned well. 'I think it's a photograph of Eddy's father, Justin,' she added.

'So that's what he looked like,' John thought, studying the picture.

'I must say that he looks remarkably like you, if you didn't have that beard,' she observed.'

'On second glance,' John said, studying the picture. 'Umm, you might be right, but as you say it's not very clear. So how did they report it? How close to what Eddy told me is it?'

John read the article.

Fire teams tackling the major blaze in the Kosciuszho National Park stumbled on to a car smash involving campers. The fire crew were alerted to an SOS sign spotted by helicopter water tankers. On arrival they discovered that the driver, Doctor Justin Jones from Sydney was seriously injured and trapped inside his crashed car. The doctor's young ten year old son, Eddy, had rendered first aid to his injured father.

The road collision occurred on a track off the main Alpine Way whilst they were apparently, looking for the Leatherbarrel creek camping ground. The pair had been trapped at the crash scene in the forest for two days and nights, following the collision with a large buck Emu.

The collision caused the driver to lose control and to slam into a tree.

Father and son were evacuated by helicopter and taken to hospital in the nick of time as the fire front quickly advanced to their location.

This paper was informed that unfortunately Doctor Jones subsequently succumbed to his injuries.

The young ten year old Eddy is being commended by the fire chief for his bravery whilst awaiting rescue, for keeping his father alive and for his quick thinking with an SOS sign which led the rescuers to their location.

'Well what do you know? Our boy's a hero,' John said, smiling.

'It's hard to reconcile that that brave ten year old is the same thirty five year old we have here, isn't it?' she observed, sadly.

'Yes. Misdiagnosed at an early age and a life lost. It truly is sad. Anyway thanks for your diligence and now I guess we should be able to plan the trip.'

'I'm on the case,' she explained.

'Thanks. In the meantime I'll see if I can track Eddy down and tell him the good news.'

John went to Eddy's house in the sheltered housing complex. Eddy came to the door at John's knock.

'Oh hello Doctor John. I wasn't expecting you. Is there something wrong. Another complaint?' he asked concerned.

'No Eddy, quite the opposite. Laura has been doing some research and has found a very interesting newspaper article about the crash.'

'Oh!' Eddy said, backing away into his house. 'I don't want to see it.'

'I think that you might like to see this, especially the bit at the end,' John informed him.

Eddy reluctantly took the article and sat down away from the Psychiatrist, he sobbed as he read it.

'So you were a hero,' John repeated, walking over to him and hugged the sobbing man. 'There you are Eddy there is no reason for you to feel bad about it, to feel guilty over. The firemen thought that you did a good job. You were a hero.'

Chapter Sixty-six

Two days later, John picked up Eddy, Marilyn, and Laura ready for the five and a half hour trip south to the Kosciuszko national park.

Eddy was still very nervous about the trip and initially reluctant to get in the car, but Marilyn kept talking at him and he soon found himself on the back seat.

'It will be lovely to see all the spring flowers coming out as we journey south,' John said, trying to cheer up the car's apprehensive passenger.

'We'll go through Sydney and along the Monaro Highway and we'll stop in Canberra for a McDonalds, how about that?'

'A McDonalds, Eddy,' Marilyn repeated gleefully. 'Did you hear, a Maccas.'

'Yes,' he replied unenthusiastically, staring blankly out of the window.

'I think we'll need the Fyshwick Exit for McDonald's then,' Laura said studying the map. '

'So everybody keep your eyes open so we don't miss it. Laura will do the navigating. But I'm sure she wouldn't mind your help, 'John suggested.

'No, I don't mind at all. I think that's a good idea,' Laura confirmed. 'Eight eyes are better than two.'

However as the journey continued, Marilyn's constant call of 'there's the exit' and 'are we nearly there yet,' soon wore thin on John and Laura's patience.

'No, it's not that one yet,' became a repeated mantra.

They had been travelling for nearly three hours before eventually they saw the Fyshwick Exit sign. By which time Marilyn had become sulky and disinterested and Eddy continued to be silent in the seat next to her.

'Here we are,' John announced. 'This is the one.'

'Thank god for that,' Laura muttered under her breath.

Marilyn suddenly became excited again. 'Is it really?' she exclaimed, staring out of the window.

'Yes, I think it's just down the road here,' John announced.

'There it is, there it is,' Marilyn squealed, spotting the famous sign after they had travelled another quarter of a mile.

John turned in to the large carpark. 'I suggest we have a break and then eat in the restaurant rather than use the drive through, I need to stretch my legs and use the toilet anyway.'

The group disembarked and went to their respective toilets.

'Eddy and I will meet you out here ladies. We're bound to be quicker than you,' John suggested, standing outside the toilet block.

John and Eddy went into the gents and, feeling slightly uncomfortable about standing next to Eddy using a urinal, John went into a cubicle and closed the door.

After he'd finished and washed his hands he went outside expecting to see Eddy already there and was surprised not to see him.

He waited a few more minutes and then went back into the toilet and got some weird looks from people as he tried all the cubicle doors, calling for Eddy.

His search was in vain, Eddy was not in the toilets.

'Oh damn,' he muttered under his breath. By the time he re-emerged from inside, Laura and Marilyn were already outside at the rendezvous point.

'Have you seen Eddy?' he asked urgently.

'No I thought he was with you,' Laura said.

'He was, but I can't find him.'

'Perhaps he's already gone into the restaurant,' Marilyn suggested. 'He eats a lot.'

John dashed into the restaurant and looked around, but no sign of Eddy.

He re-joined the ladies. 'No not in there.'

'What about the car, perhaps he's gone back there?'

John dashed off and checked.

'No, he's not there either. We need to search the area. I know he wasn't happy about the trip, but I thought with Marilyn on board he was going to man up.'

After ten minutes searching the industrial park Laura found Eddy hiding behind an advertising hoarding.

'Oh there you are. Were you playing hide and seek with us Eddy?' she said calmly.

'I don't want to go to that place. I'm scared,' Eddy muttered.

'That's why I'm here,' Marilyn explained, catching up with them. 'I'll protect you. Come on Eddy, I'm starving.'

She grabbed hold of his hand and dragged a reluctant Eddy back to the restaurant to where John had just returned.

'Ok Eddy, let's have some food. You'll feel much better when you've eaten,' John encouraged.

After a big burger meal washed down by iced coke, they returned to the car. Again Eddy was reluctant to get back in the car.

'I don't want to go,' he moaned. 'Can't we go back home now?'

'Why Eddy? We're halfway there now,' John said quietly.

'I'm scared of what we'll find,' he whined.

Marilyn grabbed hold of Eddy's hand. 'It's Ok Eddy. If John says it's going to be Ok. It will be,' she encouraged and forced him into the car with a mighty shove.

Ensuring Eddy's door was locked with the child lock, preventing him from opening it and escaping, they set off again.

'Right folks, we're almost halfway there,' Laura informed them. 'We'll re-join the main highway here and follow the B23 and B72,' she informed a disinterested audience. 'At the moment we're just on the outskirts of Canberra and we might be able to see the grand parliament buildings as we go.'

'Where?' Marilyn asked, sliding forward on the seat.

'Over there, to our right hand side.'

'I can't see it. I can't see it,' became Marilyn's new mantra. After ten minutes she eventually gave up and slumped back miserably in her seat.

'You alright Eddy?' John asked, looking at his glum face in the rear view mirror.

Eddy said nothing and continued to stare at his hands.

John and Laura exchanged looks. John was having second thoughts about his plan.

'Perhaps the trip might make things worse, rather than helping Eddy. Is there any point going on?' he thought. 'Or is it already a lost cause? Perhaps the Professor was right after all. Too late now,' he thought. 'We've come too far.'

Laura was regretting her decision to go on the trip too. The occupants weren't providing much of a stimulating atmosphere, so she decided to break the silence.

'Did you know that the Kosciuszko national park we're going to has got the highest mountain in Australia?' she informed the silent car.

'No,' Marilyn said, showing a small element of interest.

'Yes, It's 7,310 feet high.'

'Is that big?' Marilyn asked.

'Yes it's very big. People go up to the top in cable cars.'

'Can we go up there?' she asked.

'I don't think we'll have time. But, we'll see.'

'Oh Ok, she said, downhearted.

'Eddy, can you remember the name of the lake where you were going fishing with your dad?' Laura asked.

Silence.

'Eddy, did you hear?' John asked, trying to engage him.' What was the name of the lake?'

'Umm…I don't know. Jin something or other,' he muttered.

'It's Lake Jindabyne.' Laura informed them. 'Tonight, we'll be staying in a motel right on the shore of the lake.'

Chapter Sixty-seven

Finally, the weary quartet reached their destination in the small lakeside town of Jindabyne, a popular all year holiday spot.

'Here we are then,' John said, turning off the main highway and driving down the access road.

'We'll be staying at the Lake Jindabyne Motel just here,' Laura said, as John pulled up outside the reception and thankfully killed the engine. 'Apparently the original town is now under the lake following the building of the Jindabyne Dam.'

'Under the lake?' Marilyn chirped up. 'What about all the poor people?'

'Oh, they would have been rehomed before they flooded the lake.'

'How did they make the lake?' Marilyn probed.

'In 1967 they put a dam across the Snowy River and it started making the lake,' Laura explained.

'Great can we go and see it?' Marilyn enthused.

'Yes in a minute,' John confirmed. 'We need to book in first.'

'I've booked three rooms, two singles and a double,' Laura explained. 'It's only a three star, so don't expect anything too luxurious.'

'I noticed that there was a restaurant, as we came off the main highway, and suggest we eat there tonight,' John proposed. 'Everyone Ok with that?'

'Yes,' Laura and Marilyn chorused.

'I know where we are. 'Eddy said softly, breaking his silence. 'Why can't we just go to the crash site?' he asked. 'We are so close.'

'I think we've all had a long day already. After driving all that way, I for one could do with a shower and a beer,' John informed him. 'Tomorrow will be quite a strain on you Eddy. I think that you need to recharge your batteries after today's episode, don't you?'

'No…I want to go now,' Eddy insisted stubbornly.

'The site will still be there tomorrow,' Laura coaxed. 'Right, I'll go and book us in at reception,' she informed them, getting out of the car, and disappearing through into the motel.

'Let's get the stuff out of the car then,' John directed.

'No…I want to go now,' Eddy repeated, not moving.

'Look…'John started to say.

But Eddy started shouting, 'I want to go now …I want to go now.'

'Ok, now calm down Eddy,' John coaxed. 'No point getting yourself in a state. Can you talk to him Marilyn, please.'

'He won't listen to me when he's having a strop,' she replied. 'Eddy SHUT UP and get out the frigging car,' she shouted pushing him.

And to their surprise, Eddy stopped shouting, but still refused to move out of the car.

'Well done. Thank you Marilyn,' John said getting out of the car himself.

He then ignored the sulking Eddy and got the luggage out of the car himself and waited for Laura to return.

Laura returned five minutes later with their room keys.

'What's the matter with Eddy?' she asked, concerned that he was still sat in the car.

'Eddy wants to go to the site now,' John informed her, wearily.

'Well, I suppose that's a bonus, he's obviously got over his reluctance to go there,' Laura observed.

'Right, lets strike while the irons hot and go,' John suddenly proposed, putting the luggage back in the car.

'At least the motel people know we've arrived,' Laura agreed.

'Ok everybody back in the car,' John directed. 'We'll go and find the accident site now. We've had a long day, but it will all be worth it, I'm sure. Tonight we'll have some food and enjoy ourselves,' he added, trying to lift the mood of the group.

Chapter Sixty-eight

The group left the motel and John steered the car west, along the Kosciuszko Road towards the narrow Alpine Way.

'I found details of the exact location, from the fire service archives. It's near the Murray Gorge. So I know exactly where we need to go,' Laura explained.

There was a brooding silence in the car, except for Laura's directions, as they drove through the dense forest along the meandering Alpine Way to the site of Eddy's nightmare.

Although weary from his long drive down, John was sensitive to and concerned about Eddy's mental state. He kept glancing in the rear view mirror at Eddy's frightened face and the obvious inner torment that he was going through.

Marilyn was sensitive to Eddy's turmoil and held his sweating hand during the ten kilometre journey.

'It's going to be alright Eddy,' she said quietly, trying to reassure him, but unsure exactly what to do.

'John, I think we're nearly there. Slow down' Laura directed. 'Yes, this is it. Turn off the Alpine way here. Down this track on the right,' she pointed.

'Ok.'

They turned off the narrow tarmac road on to a rutted gravel track

The atmosphere in the car became tense.

'According to the faxed directions on this map, it's along here on this fire break, a few hundred yards on the left.'

After a few more minutes bouncing up and down the terracing on the track, Laura instructed him to stop. 'I think that this is it,' she revealed.

John pulled up and switched off the engine.

'Right. We're here Eddy.' John said, swivelling in his seat. 'Take your time. When you're ready, you can go to where you think you need to be. Don't worry if you can't find the exact spot. It was a long time ago and the forest has obviously healed itself. After the fire, things will look different anyway.'

'Ok,' Eddy said quietly, looking up from gazing at his lap, his heart in overdrive. He was petrified that the spectres of the past were waiting to invade his brain.

Marilyn squeezed his hand again to reassure him.

'Don't worry if you can't go any further. To be in the vicinity of where it happened will be enough for the exercise to be successful,' John explained, quietly.

After a few moments, Eddy looked around at his surroundings. Nothing frightening happened.

He reached for the door handle, and slowly opened the car door. With great trepidation, he climbed out and stood by the side of the car, initially afraid to leave his escape pod.

Slowly he looked around the small clearing, fearful of what nightmares would emerge to haunt him.

The others climbed out too and watched as Eddy slowly moved away from the car to a nearby tree. It had a piece of bark missing near the bottom of the trunk. His eyes fixed on it. Staring.

As Eddy approached the tree, his foot crunched on some broken glass hidden by the sparse undergrowth.

Immediately he knew that it was the right place. This was the windscreen glass from his father's car. It was the same glass that he had walked over, all those years before, when he ran looking for help.

He froze, as if he were stepping through a minefield. Not wishing to put another foot forward in case that would summon the horrors of the past.

Eddy's mind was suddenly deluged by a kaleidoscope of images from that appalling time when he was ten; the emu, the blood, the impact of the car hitting the tree, his father bleeding, the agonised moaning, the flies.

He felt giddy. He swayed and thought he was going to pass out and fall over, but John had been shadowing him and rushed to his aid.

Eddy put his hands over his ears to block out the dreadful wailing that echoed around the clearing. He failed to recognise that the sorrowful sound was his own hysterical voice.

His head ached as if it was going to explode. He was desperate to get away from the conjured up images from long ago. He looked around wild-eyed. He needed to escape from the bad memories rising from the cauldron of fear.

Then suddenly, he was running, running away, running down the track, away from that awful place, frightened at the prospect of opening anymore of pandora's box.

Chapter Sixty-nine

Eddy ran frantically for several hundred yards, pursued by those terrifying memories, as if the devil himself was chasing him.

He ran until he was exhausted and could run no more. His energy completely depleted, he slowly ground to a halt until he finally stopped, lungs gasping for air, his head pounding. He bent double and leant his head against a nearby tree.

Over the roaring in his ears and his frantically beating heart, he heard footsteps approaching, coming towards him.

It was his worst nightmare. Had the demons tracked him down? He eventually forced himself to look and was preparing to run again. Then to his relief John appeared.

'Flipping heck Eddy! I didn't realise you could run so fast,' John panted. 'I thought I was reasonably fit, but after fifty yards, you left me for dead.'

'I can't do it John. Please don't make me,' Eddy pleaded. 'I don't want to go back there.'

'No, of course not. It's your decision, I won't make you. You've done well to come this far. You should be proud of yourself.'

'I'm so confused. I don't know what I want,' Eddy confessed, still leaning heavily against the tree.

'That's to be expected. Your mind has hidden this trauma for a very long time and it must be an awful shock to relive it now.'

'Yes, it is. I keep having flash backs of things that happened.'

'I know, and I appreciate what a nightmare it is for you. Come on, let's go back to the car and we'll leave if you want.'

'It was…it was like stepping back in time. I remembered it all. Right back to the collision. As if I was ten again. In my mind's eye I saw the Emu appear, heard the thud and the windscreen caving in and injuring Dad. I felt the awful collision as we hit the tree. It was my fault that we hit the emu.'

'But you weren't driving. How was it your fault?'

'Because I kept telling Dad to go faster, to make the car do bigger leaps down the terracing.'

'No, you can't blame yourself for that,' John said quietly, realising that as well as the trauma of the accident, Eddy had loaded himself up with a guilty conscience believing that he had caused the accident.

'I had flashbacks of my father trapped in the car,' Eddy continued. 'The blood, the smell, the flies. The feeling of helplessness as I waited desperately for someone to come and help us. The fearful apprehension as the flames from the forest fire got closer and closer. The smoke getting thicker and thicker all the time,' Eddy relayed, surprisingly eloquently.

'That's incredible that you have remembered all that detail. Your account ties up with what you told me under hypnosis. I think that you have made the major step that I was hoping for.' John explained.

'Do you think so?'

'Yes. Just for you to make this pilgrimage was very brave. I appreciate the intensity of the emotional build up that you've gone through,' John admitted. 'You have done so well. Better than I expected.'

'Really?'

'Yes, most definitely. Come on, Let's go back to the car. The others will be concerned.'

As they re-entered the place where the car was parked, the glass, from his father's broken car windscreen, again crunched under his feet.

A chill ran through his body at the sound. Although the forest had reclaimed the area, the windscreen glass was a permanent memorial to the horrors of that day.

In spite of his earlier reluctance to revisit the memories of that awful moment, abruptly he was again transported back through the years.

He was inexplicably drawn to that particular tree, his whole body shaking as he got closer to it. Then he realised that it was the very tree that they'd crashed into. The missing piece of bark evidence of the car's impact.

Stopping directly in front of the tree, Eddy put his hand out and stroked the trunk, as if comforting a pet.

He studied the rugby ball shaped section of missing bark where the car had impacted. His fingers tracing around the smooth edges of the twelve inch scar where the tree hadn't been able to heal itself. It was an open sore.

The intimacy of the moment, connecting him back through time to the tree's witness of the devastating events of those many years past, triggered an horrendous and soulful cry. Eddy collapsed to his knees and put his arm around the tree, hugging it and resting his head against it as he wept.

Marilyn started to go to him, to comfort him, but John held her back.

'Leave him Marilyn, he needs to do this on his own, as he did all those years ago.'

'Hopefully, this is the real start of his road to recovery,' John thought. 'He's visited his demons and released the pent up guilt and fear. By the time we get back home, he should be over the initial trauma from revisiting his past.'

Slowly Eddy's sobbing abated and John went and knelt by him.

'Ok Eddy?' he asked gently, putting his arm around the other's shoulders.

'Yes, I think so,' he replied quietly.

Out of the corner of his eye, John spotted something in the undergrowth behind the base of the tree. He rummaged through the thick vegetation and picked up a small aluminium metal plate. He recognised it straightaway and showed it to Eddy.

'Do you recognise this?' John asked.

'Yes. It's… It's my dad's car number plate,' Eddy's face lit up in a broad smile. He took it reverently from John and kissed it.

'Dad was very proud of his car,' Eddy said, wiping a tear with the back of his hand. 'He had a Holden Brabham Torana with the Sports package. It used to go really fast,' he said affectionately.

'I'm glad that you will have something as a keepsake from your visit,' John smiled. 'Anyway, we'll leave you with your thoughts Eddy, while we go for a short walk, we won't be rushing back. So take your time.'

John stood up and went over to where Marilyn and Laura were standing.

'Come along ladies, we'll leave Eddy for a bit.'

'We'll see you shortly Eddy,' John called as he led the ladies down the track.

But Eddy was already talking to the numberplate, as if he were talking to his late father.

Chapter Seventy

The trio walked away from Eddy affording him some space to reflect on the life changing events of the past.

'I know that a very long time ago Eddy was involved in a crash,' Marilyn said. 'And his dad died. But why did we come here if there is nothing to see?' she puzzled.

'Yes, you're right it was many years ago and the memories have been haunting Eddy for a long time, which is why he has been poorly.

Eddy and his dad were on a fishing trip here when the accident happened. They were rescued just in time as a forest fire swept towards them,' John explained. 'Bringing him back here I hope will start to make him better. But he will have sad moments while he remembers the horrible things that happened.' John explained. 'And you can help when he is feeling sad. Will you do that Marilyn?'

'Yes of course. Eddy is my friend. The only person that likes me. All the others ignore me,' she confessed.

'I'm sure that's not true,' Laura said, putting her arm around Marilyn's shoulders. 'What do you think about this lovely forest? Isn't it gorgeous in its spring finery?

'Yes, looking at the forest now you wouldn't know that all these trees would have been burnt so badly, would you?' John pointed out.

The mention of fire had a strange effect on Marilyn, she suddenly started shaking as if she was about to fit.

'But Eddy escaped from the fire didn't he?' Marilyn sought confirmation, her eyes staring.

'Yes he did. But are you alright?' John asked, concerned.

The group stopped, John and Laura looked anxiously at Marilyn.

'It's been a long day, she's probably overtired,' Laura suggested.

'My people didn't escape,' Marilyn revealed, in a haunting voice.

'Oh, that's terribly sad. I'm sorry to hear that,' Laura sympathised but not really understanding what Marilyn was talking about.

'But I didn't mean for it to happen,' Marilyn muttered, staring wide-eyed at the floor.

John and Laura exchanged concerned glances but said nothing.

After a few minutes Marilyn came out of her 'episode' and they continued their walk.

'Obviously, some trauma there that needs to be investigated when we get back,' John thought.

After the others had left him, Eddy sat with his back to the tree, hugging the number plate to his chest. Slowly all the memories of his childhood started filtering back, populating his mind.

He smiled and cried as he battled the fog in his head while he remembered all the pleasant things that he'd done with his dad, fishing, swimming, first aid, meeting people.

And then he burst in to tears as he recalled the dreadful, life shattering message at the hospital that his dad was dead.

'Remember Eddy, your fast thinking extended your dad's life,' the nurse had told him. *'In the end his injuries were too severe so that not even the expert doctors could save him. I am sure that your dad was very proud of what you did.'*

Consequently, half an hour later as the others re-joined him, he had relived the rollercoaster of emotions associated with his dad and although sad, he was feeling a lot better.

Eddy had made a small cross from sticks and intertwined it with some of the undergrowth and laid it against the tree.

'That's nice,' Marilyn said, looking at Eddy's tribute.

'Thank you,' he said.

'If you are happy Eddy, I think we've done what I wanted you to achieve, let's go.'

'Yes. I feel a lot better thank you.'

'Come on then people,' John directed.

The others climbed back into the car, but before getting in, Eddy gave the tree a final hug and whispered, 'I love you Dad.'

With tears in his eyes, he climbed back into the car still hugging the number plate that John had found.

Chapter Seventy-one

The trip back from the crash site to the motel was quiet. Each lost in their own thoughts. The others were all sensitive to the ordeal that Eddy had gone through.

On their return to the motel, Laura dug out the room keys that she'd got earlier.

They silently unloaded their bags and made their way together to the corridor linking all their rooms.

Laura opened her and John's room and they deposited their overnight bags in to the sparsely decorated room and returned to the others.

'We'll help you two with opening your rooms,' John offered. 'Oh by the way, I suggest we all go together to the restaurant later,' he added.

'What time?' Laura asked.

'Let's say seven o'clock. Out front by the car,' he suggested.

'Let's get you into your rooms first then. Marilyn, you are next door in room five,' Laura said, leading Marilyn to the small room.

'Thank you. I...I've never stayed in a Motel before,' Marilyn said apprehensively. 'What do I have to do?'

'It's just like living in your own house,' John explained. 'It's a room where you can rest, bathe and sleep.'

'Don't worry, I'll help you,' Laura said.

'I'll help Eddy,' John volunteered. 'Eddy, here's your room, it's number four,' he said, checking his key.

All the rooms were en-suite with a shower cubical in the corner of the small bathroom. The bedroom was neat, clean, and basically equipped with a bed, a small wardrobe, and a dressing table with a set of drawers.

Each room had a large sliding French window which gave access to the small patio from which there were wonderful views over the lake. A small air conditioning unit stood outside each room next to a table and chair.

Marilyn was excited as Laura opened the door.

'Is this all mine?' she asked enthusiastically.

'Yes, all yours for tonight,' Laura confirmed.

Marilyn rushed around the room like an overjoyed child, checking the bathroom, turning on the shower and bouncing on the bed.

Meanwhile, next door, John opened the door for a subdued Eddy.

'Here you are Eddy, this is your room.'

'Thank you,' he said softly, walking in and sitting on the bed, still clutching the number plate.

'You've had a bit of an ordeal today Eddy. I suggest that you have a doze,' John advised. 'We've got an hour or so before we go to the restaurant.'

Eddy lay back on the bed and closed his eyes, cradling the number plate to his chest.

'You did brilliantly today Eddy,' John praised his patient. 'I am very pleased the way that you coped with it. It will get better from now on, you see,' John reassured him, and left Eddy alone with his thoughts, closing the door quietly behind him.

As he left Eddy's room, John's pager buzzed as a new message came in.

'Bugger, I thought I'd switched that off,' he thought, looking at the message.

'How long before I get the information or I visit the police?'

'Bitch,' John muttered under his breath.

Annoyed at the intrusion, he made his way to join Laura in their room.

'What's up John? she asked, seeing his glum face.

'Somehow that bitch has got my pager number. And she's chasing me for an answer,' he explained.

'Oh no! Well the only way she could get that is from me or my relief in the office. The Professor hasn't got it,' she explained. 'I certainly wouldn't give it out.'

'Well, she's got it now,' John said angrily.

'What are you going to do?' Laura asked, concerned.

'Ignore her until I get back. In the mean time I'll switch the thing off,' John said, sliding the pager switch to the off position.

Chapter Seventy-two

After a quick cup of tea and a refreshing shower John and Laura rustled up Eddy and Marilyn.

Eddy had gone to sleep on the bed and hadn't changed, Marilyn had had a shower and a bath, such was the novelty of having her own room.

The group made their way on foot to the nearby Banjo Paterson restaurant for their evening meal.

'Well done today Eddy. In the morning we'll have breakfast and a leisurely trip back home, perhaps even doing some sightseeing on the way,' John suggested.

'Sightseeing! Yeah,' Marilyn said, enthusiastically.

They arrived at the smart looking restaurant and as they opened the door a waiter was quickly at their side.

'Good evening. Were you thinking of dining tonight?' he asked.

'Yes please. Could we have a table for four.'

'Yes of course, please follow me,' the waiter said, leading them to a large circular table, before handing each one a menu.

Unaccustomed to dining out, Eddy and Marilyn took theirs and looked at it blankly. Wondering what it was for.

'Don't worry,' John reassured them. We'll do the ordering; in the meantime do you want a drink?'

'Yes please, they chorused.

'Do you sell beer here?' John asked

'Yes,' the waiter confirmed.

In finally agreeing for Eddy and Marilyn to go on the trip, the Professor insisted that they should not be given any alcohol.

When John challenged the Professor on his ruling, he said that several contraindications show an adverse effect to people on the trial where alcohol was used. However, ignoring the Professors words of caution, and as he adjudged the day a success, John decided that a small beer wouldn't 'harm' and he decided to risk it.

'Four bottles of low alcohol beer, please,' John asked.

Marilyn giggled like an excited school girl at the prospect of having a beer, the 'forbidden fruit'.

'I'll leave you with the menu,' the waiter said, leaving to get their drinks.

Laura took charge of ordering from the menu.

'So people what do we want? To start there's Soup or a Fish dish?

'Although I used to go fishing. I remember that I didn't like eating fish,' Eddy volunteered. 'Could I have the soup please?'

'Me too,' Marilyn added.

'Ok, now the main dish. It's lots of different seafood; Beef; Lamb or Kangaroo.'

'Kangaroo! ' Marilyn repeated in surprise. 'Oh I don't think so.'

'You would have to hop around chasing it with your knife and fork,' Eddy observed, laughing.

'Oh he's brightening up at last,' John thought.

'No you wouldn't Marilyn,' said innocently. 'It would be dead.'

'How about a beef steak?' John suggested. 'With shoestring fries?'

'Yes please,' Eddy and Marilyn chorused.

'I shall have the Wok Tossed Tofu.' Laura said. 'I quite like a vegetarian meal occasionally.'

'Ok. What about Ice cream for dessert?' John asked.

'Yes please,' was the group's unanimous agreement.

So when the waiter brought their drinks and distributed the bottles of beer, John was able to give him the food order.

John poured his beer carefully in to the glass which had already been laid out on the table. Eddy and Marilyn however, decided to drink out of the bottle. Laura followed John's example.

'Well done everyone, I think it's been a successful trip,' John toasted, lifting his glass to 'chink' with the others.

As they waited for their food to arrive they discussed the wonderful scenery that they had witnessed as they had driven to their location; the magnificent forests, the fast-flowing rivers, and the big dam just outside the town.

'It is lovely, but I miss the sea,' Marilyn giggled, clearly showing the early effects of the beer.

Eventually the meal arrived and they all tucked in. Eddy had now joined Marilyn in demonstrating some boisterous tipsy behaviour.

Having refused several requests from his patients for more beer. John was happy to pay the bill and quickly leave.

'The Professor was obviously right about restricting the booze,' he thought as he and Laura carefully shepherded the singing duo of Eddy and Marilyn back to the motel.

Eventually they managed to get the raucous pair into their respective rooms. They had to foil several attempts where the pair wanted to 'escape' and go down to the lake. However they were finally persuaded to stay in their rooms.

'Goodnight Eddy, good night Marilyn. We'll see you in the morning.'

However, before turning in themselves and in order to ensure that their charges stayed in their rooms, John and Laura sat outside Eddy and Marilyn's rooms until their charges went quiet.

After half an hour 'on guard', the pair finally turned in themselves and had been in bed for only ten minutes when Laura heard shouting outside.

Chapter Seventy-three

Laura woke John. 'John, John. What's all that noise?' she asked.

'Oh god, what are those two up to now? Perhaps the Prof was right about avoiding alcohol.'

They quickly threw on some clothes and ran to the source of the noise which they discovered was coming from the lake.

Then they spotted them. Both of them were in the water, but Marilyn was further out and clearly in distress. She kept disappearing under the water as Eddy was swimming towards her.

'Oh shit!' John said, diving in to the lake. As he swam towards them, both Eddy and Marilyn disappeared under the water.

John increased his frantic stroke rate to reach where he'd last seen them. Behind him he heard Laura dive in as well.

He was ten yards from where he judged they had disappeared when suddenly both heads resurfaced.

Eddy was on his back and had Marilyn in a rescue hold supporting her chin out of the water. Eddy, started swimming effortlessly with his casualty back to the shore.

Meanwhile Laura joined John.

'Are they alright?' she asked, treading water.

'Not sure about Marilyn, but Eddy seems to know what he's doing,' John replied.

John was going to take over the rescue, but could see that Eddy had things under control, so he swam alongside them, just in case he was needed.

When they got to shallow water, they took the unconscious woman out of the lake. John lifted Marilyn's feet while Eddy carried her under her armpits and laid her down on the grass bank

Marilyn was wearing her nightie, and Eddy was in his pyjamas.

Eddy immediately started pumping Marilyn's chest and after a few minutes she showed signs of life, she stirred and vomited lake water. Eddy quickly turned her on her side as she continued to be sick.

'Content with Eddy's obvious command of the situation, John just carefully monitored Marilyn's vital signs.'

A group of other motel guests gathered round them, attracted by the shouting.

A concerned resident asked 'Are they Ok? Should I call for an ambulance?'

'No, it's Ok,' John explained. 'I'm a doctor. I'll deal with it, but thanks anyway.'

Eddy was clearly exhausted by his rescue and resuscitation efforts and sat back on his haunches panting.

'Well done Eddy. You saved her life. Are you Ok?'

'Yes,' he wheezed.

'I didn't know that you knew about lifesaving and resuscitation,' Laura observed.

'I...I think that I must have always known it. That's right...now I think about it. My Dad insisted on me doing it,' he revealed. 'He said...said, if we were going to be near water doing fishing, I...I had to know how to do these things,' Eddy expanded.

'Memory recall is continuing,' John thought, pleased at seeing Eddy's progress. 'A very good sign that the trip had been well worth the risk.'

'That's weird. Until now, I had never remembered that,' Eddy said realising more snatches of his childhood were coming back to him.

Marilyn stirred and propped herself up on one elbow.

'Ok Marilyn?' John asked.

'Yes,' she coughed and belched loudly; which brought nervous laughter from the rescuers.

'What were you doing in the lake at this time of night, anyway?' he continued

'I had a nightmare. I was escaping from my burning house. My clothes were on fire. I had to put them out.' Marilyn whispered hoarsely.

'I thought you could swim Marilyn?' Laura questioned.

'I can, but I must have been dreaming and the cold water woke me up. I didn't know where I was, so I panicked,' she revealed.

'I heard her shouting and then I heard her open the outside door,' Eddy explained. 'I wondered what was happening. I tried talking to her but she didn't reply. She was running. I followed her all the way down to the lake trying to get her to speak. I couldn't believe it when she just ran in,' he informed them. 'Then she started flailing around calling for help. So I just went in after her.'

'Eddy's my hero. You saved me again,' Marilyn said, hugging him.

'I did, didn't I?' he beamed.

'You should be very proud of yourself Eddy. Your quick actions definitely saved Marilyn's life.'

'Eddy, you rescued me. Didn't you?' Marilyn repeated.

'I had to. You're my best friend,' Eddy said, squeezing her.

'Come on then you two. Let's get you out of those wet things,' John said, helping Marilyn to her feet.

As they walked back to their rooms, Laura walked alongside Marilyn, as Eddy supported her.

Chapter Seventy-four

The following morning John went to raise Eddy and Marilyn for breakfast but found their rooms empty.

'Oh shit, now where are they?' he panicked. After the midnight swimming drama, I hope they haven't been up to any mischief.'

John wandered around the site anxiously looking for the pair. Then he heard some excited voices coming from near the water's edge. The voices were interspersed with splashes and cheering.

'Surely they're not swimming in the lake again,' he thought.

He increased his pace and as he rounded the end of the building, to his relief he could see that the pair were together on the bank, throwing stones in to the lake.

'Thank God for that,' he thought.

'Good morning you two. Are you ready for breakfast?' John asked, relieved to have found them.

'Yes please,' they chorused.

'We'll just pick up Laura on the way to the café, 'he informed them. 'How did you sleep after last night's adventures?'

'I just went to sleep like normal,' Marilyn said, surprised at the question.

'Eddy, what about you?' John quizzed.

'Oh very well thanks,' Eddy lied.

'Are you sure? You look a bit…a bit tired to me,' John observed. 'I wouldn't be surprised if you had a poor night after your lifesaving efforts.'

'No, it wasn't that. I kept thinking about 'things' again. You know…from my childhood.'

'It's only to be expected. There are so many things stored in the hidden places of your mind that your memory will continue to recall,' John reassured him. 'I'm sure that you will start to feel so much better, soon. Trust me.'

'Ok, if you say so.'

'Don't worry Eddy. I won't let anything hurt you,' Marilyn said, putting her arm round his shoulders. 'You're my hero.'

'I hope you're right Marilyn,' John thought. 'Now we've opened the flood gates, who knows how the spectres of the past will affect him? I just hope my gambling with his psyche will pay off long term.'

Having collected Laura, the group went to the nearby café and had a full Australian breakfast.

'Is Eddy Ok John?' Laura asked as they walked back to the car. 'He looks a bit tired and was unusually quiet over breakfast. Was it anything to do with last night's drama?'

'No, he says not. Although he's a bit short on sleep, he reckons it's because his memories are flooding back. But he'll be Ok, I hope.' John explained. 'My concern now is Marilyn. We've obviously woken something up in her past too, that concerns me.'

'Yes likewise. I don't know her history, only that she is a bit of a brawler and if there's a punch up, she's usually the cause of it.'

'When we get back, I'll add her to my case load. Did you give them their pills that the Professor insisted they take?'

'Yes, but I'm not sure that they took them,' Laura confessed.

'Oh well, we tried,' John said flippantly. 'In any case, I'll definitely get Eddy removed from the trial so he'll stand a chance of repairing the brain damage caused by decades of mistreatment.'

Chapter Seventy-five

Having collected their overnight bags and waited for John to pay for their accommodation, the group left the motel and headed back along the Kosciuszko Road heading for home.

They spent some time visiting the huge great dam complex, which had created lake Jindabyne.

At Marilyn's insistence, the quartet took the 15 minutes scenic ride on the Kosciuszko Express Chairlift to the summit. 'You promised,' she reminded Laura.

The ride offered breathtaking views of the Kosciuszko National Park and the stunning Thredbo Valley as it rose 560 vertical metres to its destination.

At the top of the mountain they wandered around the usual tourist shops looking at various tourist memorabilia. Marilyn was particularly taken by some glass paperweights containing images of the mountain and it's slopes.

'Can I please have one of these?' she asked John.

'Have you got any money?' he asked, already knowing the answer.

'No. I haven't,' Marilyn said despondently.

'Don't worry, Marilyn. I will buy it for you,' Laura said generously. 'Did you want one as well Eddy?'

'No thanks. I have my Dad's number plate to remind me of the trip,' he explained.

'OK, just Marilyn's then.'

Laura paid and gave the paperweight to Marilyn.

'Thank you Laura, this will help me when I'm feeling sad.'

While they were at the top of the mountain, they even checked out the start of some of the hiking trails that crisscrossed the mountainside.

'It would be lovely to go for a walk up here,' John said. 'Sadly, we have to be heading for home.'

'Can we have some lunch first?' Marilyn asked.

'OK, I suppose we might as well,' he agreed.

Finally satisfied that they'd seen enough, John treated them all to lunch at Eagles Nest, Australia's highest restaurant.

The group caught the chairlift down, admiring all the magnificent views of forest and mountains as they descended.

'Well that was good fun, wasn't it?' Laura said, as they returned to the car.

'It was just what the doctor ordered after the tensions of the previous day,' John thought. 'A good relaxer.'

'Right, as we didn't see it on the way down we'll pop into the Snowy Hydro Discovery Centre on the way back. We'll probably all need to use the toilet by then,' John said as they pulled out of the carpark.

Several hours later they pulled into the Discovery Centre car park.

'Everybody awake?' John asked the quiet car.

'That drive after a lovely lunch sent us all off to sleep,' Laura yawned, stretching.

'Just as well that I stayed awake then,' John pointed out.

'You're our hero,' Laura mocked.

'This bit of fresh air should soon wake us up again. I could do with a coffee to keep myself awake for the final bit of the journey home,' John explained.

'What is this place,' Eddy asked sleepily, looking around.

'According to the poster, the Snowy Hydro centre is a dynamic energy company. It's one of the largest electricity generators in the National Electricity Market,' John informed him.

'How does it do that?' Marilyn asked.

'It uses the force of the water to turn turbines and these turn generators which make electricity, John explained.

'Oh is that all?' Marilyn said, disinterested in the explanation.

The group spent an hour there having a coffee and exploring the facilities.

At John's insistence, the last thing they did was to visit the toilets before heading for home. This time Eddy did not run and hide.

'Right, next stop home I think,' John said, checking the fuel gauge. I'm glad that I filled up in town before we left this morning.'

During the trip home Eddy slept erratically, his memory awakened. The likeness of John to his father now causing Eddy to feel uneasy.

Meanwhile, as they got closer to Manly, John's thoughts strayed to the blackmail threats from

Sophie Mcbid. He was getting more and more anxious about her dreadful allegations and what he should do about them. He could find no answer to his dilemma.

Chapter Seventy-six

After a good night's sleep John reluctantly switched his pager back on. Immediately it bleeped with another message from Sophie.

'Time is running out. Call me urgently.'

'Bitch,' he fumed. But she'll have to wait for a bit longer. I need to sort out Eddy first'.

John went to the Professor's office to give his report in about the trip and his intentions of 'rescuing' Eddy from his involvement in the trial.

'Hello John, come in and take a seat. Well, how did it go?' the other demanded, smugly, expecting a disastrous report.

'Yes it went well. Absolutely fine,' John beamed. 'It went even better than I was expecting.'

'Really?'

'Yes it appears that my gamble has paid off. Eddy is now going through the various stages of memory recall and as such I'd like to withdraw him from your trial.'

'Withdraw him! We've already had this discussion. Why nothings changed?'

'A great deal has changed. This is to enable him to recover in a drug free regime,' he told the astonished academic.

'Absolutely not. As I've said before he is an integral part of my trial. To withdraw him now will cause a significant distortion of the results,' the Professor said vehemently.

'But I think whatever medication that he is now on is actually holding back his complete recovery,' John pleaded.

'The trial is bigger than one individual,' the academic said angrily. 'The study results will be scrutinised internationally. It will be significant in providing evidence for my theory of a complete cure for mental illness. I won't jeopardise my results by allowing any intrusion to the controlled group of patients.'

'Eddy is my patient and I insist he is withdrawn from the trial,' John said firmly. 'With or without your permission.'

'Absolutely not. Please remember to whom you are talking.'

'Or is it something more to do with hiding the real facts about the casualty toll of your trial?

'What?'

'And a cosy financial relationship with the drug company, rather than seeking a true scientific result?' John suggested awkwardly.

'What? What are you suggesting? I don't believe what I've just heard,' the Professor protested, flabbergasted.

'I've seen documents that seem to suggest that a lot of people have died after taking part in the trial. In addition you are getting a kickback from the drug firm. Therefore you are deliberately producing false evidence to prove that the drugs are working, when in fact they aren't.' John accused, feeling uncomfortable at making the allegations.

'How dare you,' the Professor challenged. 'Are you out of your mind? Where has this pack of fiction come from?'

'I'm sorry, I can't tell you my sources. However if you allow Eddy to come off the trial, then I shall withdraw my comments.'

'Withdraw your comments! Don't you dare blackmail me with your nonsensical gossip. I am surprised and disappointed at your lack of propriety.'

'Likewise, when I learned that a respected academic like yourself would appear to be running an unauthorised trial and forging results and taking bribes.'

'I refute your vile allegations. The paper that I'm writing will see a whole mind shift away from conventional thinking. I am not going to allow some pathetic hypnotherapist to spoil all my work. Do you hear me?' the Professor demanded. 'Eddy Jones stays on my trial. Now I suggest you leave my office and reconsider your position here.'

John was surprised at the Professor's unwavering refusal to withdraw Eddy from the trial. Even the revelation from Sophie about the hidden deaths had not been enough to make him change his mind. John was now feeling decidedly uncomfortable about having repeated Sophie's allegations. Had the cursed reporter 'set him up' in order to falsely discredit the Professor?

Chapter Seventy-seven

John was frustrated by being unable to reach an amicable arrangement with the Professor about withdrawing Eddy from the trial. He was further disappointed in himself at allowing Sophie Mcbid's unfounded threats to undermine his own professionalism.

He moped about in the office doing unproductive work until it was time to go home. Still beating himself up he returned to his apartment.

To his surprise, Laura greeted him as he entered the flat.

'Hello handsome, I left work early and I've made a salad for tea.' she smiled, kissing and hugging him. He did not respond.

Alerted by his unresponsive body language she stepped back and looked into his eyes. 'Oh dear by the look on your face something's wrong.'

'Yes, the Professor isn't going to withdraw Eddy from the trial,' John informed her.

'But surely that's no surprise to you? He's invested a lot of time in his trial.'

'No, I suppose not. But I was hoping to persuade him.'

'How?'

'That woman and her death certificates. I got annoyed and used the accusations that that woman fed me. I shouldn't have done that with unsubstantiated allegations, especially as it came from her. I am gutted that I even undermined my own scruples.'

'No you shouldn't, you're right. These journalists use false information all the time to winkle out secrets.'

And worse still, the chances of getting any more useful information from the Professor to handover to her is now virtually nil. Especially as I've just accused him of falsifying the casualty rate and cosying up to the drug company to hide it. I've just criticised his trial as a fraud.'

'What! Are you out of your mind? Why did you do that? So what are you going to do now?' she asked.

'I don't know. I should report her to the police. On the other hand, I can't let that woman's false rape accusations ruin my career,' John said firmly.

'Well short of 'knocking her off', you'll just have to give her any information that you know about the Professor's trial,' Laura said, emphatically.

'I know, but even though we have fallen out about Eddy I can't do that to him. I'd be the assassin of his professional career. The guy was good enough to employ me. I can't stab him in the back for this bitch,' John reasoned.

'Well it's either him or you,' Laura pointed out.

'I know but...'

'If only you had some evidence to prove your innocence.' Laura suggested.

'Yes, I know that...but what? It's my word against hers and with that condom she has forensic evidence on her side. Albeit fixed.'

John wandered over to gaze out of the window, desperately looking for inspiration, Laura followed him. As she did so, her eye was drawn to the phone.

'What's this flashing light on your phone John?' Laura asked.

'I don't know. I'm not into techie things,' John confessed. 'It's been on for a few days, maybe weeks. I don't know. It's not going to help me sort this mess out though is it?'

'I think it's showing that there's a recording on it,' Laura said, studying the telephone carefully.

'Well I haven't been recording anything,' John advised her.

'Are you sure?'

'I didn't even know that it had that facility.'

'I reckon if we press this…button labelled playback,' she said pressing it.

The telephone started playing a recording that John was very pleased to hear.

'There's your lifesaver John,' Laura said to her delighted boyfriend.

Chapter Seventy-eight

Sophie was called back to the production office and knocked on the Producer's door. She entered and was surprised to see John sitting by the side of the Producer.

'Come in, sit down Sophie. I believe you know John Masters here?' the Producer said stiffly.

'Yes, I do. Nice to meet you again John,' she lied, her heart going ninety to the dozen.

Sophie sat down, apprehensive of why the meeting had been called.

'How are your investigations into the mental health scandal going?' the Producer asked casually.

'Fine. John is going to help me with the fine detail. Isn't that right John?' she asked.

'Yes. But not in the way that you expect,' John smiled. 'Allow me to play this recording for you and I think it will help.' John pressed some buttons on his tape recorder and adjusted the volume. Sophie's voice came from the tiny speaker.

'Don't you remember? Yes when I came to seek help because my car had broken down. You raped me.'

'You are deluded. Where has this come from? You know that's not true.'

'Yes, I know that but the police don't. And as a victim they will believe me. Especially when they find your semen on my clothes.'

'Semen! I've never been anywhere near you.'

'No, but your poor housekeeping leaving used condoms on the bedroom floor will help me prove my case.'

Sophie's heart stopped. The game was up.

John switched the phone recording off and looked at her sternly.

'What have you got to say Sophie?' the Producer demanded.

'Well I…Of course I was never going to do that. No of course not. I…mean …I just wanted to flush out the scandal at the hospital, that's all. I think the ends justified the means,' she blustered.

'Accusing someone of rape! Threatening to ruin their reputation, their lives. Of course it doesn't. You have crossed the line this time,' the Producer shouted angrily. 'You are fired.'

'I was only trying to do what you wanted. You wanted a scoop, I was going to give you a scoop,' she screeched.

'A scoop, yes. But not like this. Using blackmail! Making false allegations!'

'I was close,' she insisted. 'I have documented evidence that the Professor was falsifying the death rate of people on the trial and he was in collusion with the Pharmaceutical company. I've copies of death certificates to prove it.'

'You're too late with that one. I've had a complaint from a graphic designer about an unpaid bill. When I asked what it was for, he told me that you got him to forge copies of death certificates and bank statements.'

'I..I only pre-empted what was probably going on in this scandalous drugs trial,' she protested.

'Probably! Probably is not a reason to make up lies. The integrity of this production company is my responsibility and by your devious actions you have undermined that.'

'But you were happy to get the ratings weren't you?'

'Within an honest environment, yes.'

'Yeah, right. You don't know the meaning of honest,' she ranted. 'You were quite happy for me to use this forged stuff in the past to flush the truth out,' she accused. 'I've worked my butt off for this company and you know it,' she seethed. 'You know how you got your viewing figures? By me putting my life on the line. Well there are other production companies that will be interested in taking me on,' she raged angrily.

'Not when I tell them of your underhand methods they won't,' the Producer retorted. 'The financial damages for libel and perjury awarded by any court could be astronomical.'

'Bastard.'

John broke his silence, gratified to hear confirmation of Sophie's conniving methods.

'I have to warn you that if I hear anything about your lies, concerning anything purported to be going on at the hospital, then this tape will go to the police,' John said calmly. 'And I'll insist that you are charged with blackmail. Do you hear?'

John picked up his tape recorder and left the television executive's office with a spring in his step.

With victory ringing in his ears, John couldn't wait to tell Laura.

Behind him Sophie 'shot daggers' at him.

'And you Mcbid can go too. We are done. NOW GET OUT,' the producer shouted angrily.

'I'm not done yet,' Sophie raged, as she stormed out of the office. 'I'll expose this cover up too. I won't be gagged. They'll be sorry.'

Chapter Seventy-nine

John had gone back to the institute and found Laura at the reception desk.

'My, look at you. What a change. You look very happy,' she said, looking up as he crossed the floor.

'Yes. Thanks to your 20 x 20 vision again spotting that recording on my telephone, that TV reporter has got the sack,' he beamed.

'Oh great. Well done you,' she chuckled.

'When I played the recording to the Producer of her trying to blackmail me he was horrified. He immediately called her into his office. You should have seen the look on her face when I played the tape. Well if looks could kill, I'd be in my box,' a jubilant John explained.

'The evil bitch got her comeuppance at last,' Laura said vociferously.

'Come here you,' he said, going around the desk and giving her a big hug. 'Thank you for your support and faith in me.'

'See, I did believe in you,' she confirmed. So is that it then?' Laura asked. Has she stopped her investigations into the Institute?'

'No, I doubt it. She'll continue to try and stitch the Professor up and sell it to another television company,

I expect. But at least she won't be threatening me anymore.'

'Should we warn the Professor?' Laura wondered.

'Yes, and I need to apologise to him too,' John said humbly.

'Yes I think so too.'

'No wonder I was fooled, that woman got a graphic designer to forge those death certificates and bank statements.'

'Is there no end to her evil ways?' Laura remarked.

'I think we'll need to keep an eye on Eddy too. He's had dealings with her and now he's having memory recall, he's psychologically vulnerable,' John observed.

'Yes, that's true.

Chapter Eighty

Sophie had left the TV Producers office seething. Her face white with rage.

'How dare he sack me!' she ranted. 'I'll show them. Nobody messes with me.'

Fortunately for her, the Producer hadn't got around to instructing the security officer to escort her off the premises, so she returned to her office still raging.

She picked up the components of her Sheila disguise and went to the ladies toilet and transformed into the anti-psychiatry protestor. I'll show them,' she said making up Sheila's face in the mirror.

'If he doesn't want to take the story, I'll sell it to the opposition,' she thought. 'If I can't get it broadcast one way, I'll get it another. I won't be defeated.'

She left the production offices for the last time and tracked Eddy down in the park near his house.

'G'day Eddy,' she said as she sidled up to him and stood close.

Having now come to terms with discovering his past life Eddy was feeling happy and delighted at her closeness. He thought it confirmed the romantic status between them.

'G'day Sheila,' Eddy beamed. 'Nice to see you,' he said, playfully punching her on the shoulder.

'Will you stop thumping me. You have the 'social skills' of a fuckin gorilla,' she said irritably.

'Oh I'm sorry. Can I give you a cuddle?' Eddy said, attempting to hug her.

'Sod off you freak,' she screeched, backing away from him.

Eddy was stunned. 'But I thought you loved me,' Eddy pleaded.

'Loved you! Yeah if you like,' she said insincerely.'

'Eddy started to put his arm around her shoulders again.

Finally, her temper exploded. All her carefully contrived pretence was shattered. 'Get off me you freak! Do you think I would possibly like you, let alone love you? 'Go back to one of your own kind, that emotional tumbleweed girlfriend of yours, that Marilyn.'

'But she is my friend not my girlfriend. I gave up my friend for you to be my girlfriend… I…'I ditched her for you.' Eddy repeated, devastated at her rejection. 'I…I… love you.' He put his head in his hands and started to sob.

'Well there you go! You're gonna have to un-ditch her then aren't you? Welcome to the world of 'hard knocks' sweetie. This is real life. Not like your cosy world of drugged euphoria. Life's a shit and the sooner you learn that, the sooner you can get off those chemical crutches,' she ranted.

'But I loved you,' he repeated sobbing. 'You said you loved me too. Now I've got nothing.'

'Grow up Eddy. I need some more information. Get it and I'll review our friendship.'

'No you can't be horrible to me. We are in love,' he pleaded.

'Love! You don't know the meaning of it,' she demeaned.

Just at that point Marilyn arrived to see a distraught Eddy.

'What's the matter Eddy,' she asked concerned.

'He wants his nappy changing,' Sophie ridiculed.

'Don't you dare talk about Eddy like that. He saved my life twice. He is my hero,' Marilyn said angrily, facing up to her.

'Hero! Ha! Yes. Captain Boohoo! Just look at him, snivelling. He's no more a hero than my little finger,' Sophie continued mocking him.

Marilyn grabbed Sophie's dress and put her face into the others. 'One more word and you'll be on your back,' she shouted.

'Touch me and you'll be locked up where all you loons should be,' Sophie seethed.

She misread the seriousness of Marilyn's bluster, but soon felt the sincerity of it seconds later as Marilyn delivered a right hook to her jaw.

Sophie, or rather Sheila as Eddy knew her, was flat on her back before she knew it, her wig falling off and false prosthetic teeth knocked out.

'Oh my god Marilyn look what you've done,' Eddy rebuked. 'You've knocked her teeth out. Now you're in trouble!'

'Here hang on Eddy,' Marilyn warned. 'There's something suspicious here. She's not who she says she is. She's that reporter lady from the television. She's been wearing a disguise. The bitch has been having you on all the time.'

Distraught at the revelation of Sophie's deception, Eddy ran away, deeply distressed.

'You vicious bitch,' Sophie said, picking herself up and going toe to toe with Marilyn ready to fight. 'You'll regret that,' she seethed.

Just at that moment Police Sergeant Jon Baldy screeched to a halt in his patrol car and seeing the two women facing up to each other rushed over.

'Right ladies, that's enough. Back off now, both of you,' he said forcing them apart. 'I've just come from the television offices looking for you Sophie.'

'Well I don't work there anymore,' she relayed angrily, still viciously maintaining eye contact with Marilyn.

'So I gathered. Now I have fingerprint evidence from the murder weapon that killed Digger Lucas.'

'I didn't kill him,' Marilyn said, fearfully, stepping away from the Policeman.

'But I warned you before about carrying a knife Marilyn, didn't I?' the Sergeant said sternly. 'But I know that you didn't kill him.'

'Oh, thank goodness,' she said, putting her hand over her fast beating heart.

'However, Sophie Mcbid I am arresting you on suspicion of murder. You have the right to remain silent. Anything you say can be used against you in court,' the Policeman said, reaching for his handcuffs whilst holding her wrist.

Sophie didn't resist. She turned to allow herself to be handcuffed.

'It was an accident,' she pleaded. 'I was after some information about the Professor and he tried to sexually assault me. He threatened me with his knife. We struggled and fell over. He fell on his own knife. I tried taking the knife out of him, but it was stuck…and that's why my fingerprints are on it.'

'Tell that to the Judge,' he said sceptically, securing the handcuffs.

'Come on Jon, we can talk about this,' Sophie said. 'I thought our little business arrangements might help sort this out…' she pleaded.

'Do you want me to add attempting to bribe an officer of the law to the charges Sophie?

'Bastard! Anyway she's the one who should be arrested and charged for assault. She punched me in the face,' the TV reporter raged.

Ignoring her accusation, the Policeman led Sophie to the Police car and closed the door.

He went back over to a confused Marilyn.

'And you Marilyn. What have I told you about fighting? You might want to put something on your knuckle it appears bruised,' he smiled, got into his car and drove his prisoner off to the police station.

Chapter Eighty-one

On returning to his office John found an official looking envelope on his desk.

He ripped it open with fevered fingers. The envelope contained certified copies of Eddy's and his own birth certificates from the UK.

With mounting excitement, the first certificate he read was Eddy's. His eyes latched on to the handwritten entries.

'Where and when born:'
Sixteenth November 1946; 14 Hatherley Road.'
'So he is two years older than me,' John observed.
Registration District; *Gloucester* Sub District; *Gloucester.*
Name; *Edward John*
Sex; *Boy*
Name and surname of father; *Justin Jones*
Mother's Name, Surname and Maiden name; *Samantha Jones formerly Masters.*

'Masters! That's a bit of a coincidence. That's the same name as my mother and I.'

Occupation of father; *Doctor*

'That's interesting. Mother's name is Masters,' he mused. Then he picked up the copy of his own birth certificate and quickly scanned it.

Where and when born.
Fifteenth July 1948; Tewkesbury Maternity hospital.'
Registration District; *Gloucester* Sub District; *Tewkesbury*
Name; *John James*
Sex; *Boy*
Name and Surname of father ; *Justin Jones.*

'What! No way! There must be some mistake!' He collapsed back in his chair in disbelief.

'This is just too much of a coincidence. I've waited years to find out who my father was. Why didn't I think of getting a copy of my birth certificate before?' John berated himself.

Mother's Name, Surname and Maiden name; *Samantha Jones formerly Masters.*

They must have got divorced. So my mother must have changed her name, our name, back to her maiden name. Well I'll be!

Occupation of father; *Doctor.*

'No this can't be right?' John slumped back in his chair again, his head in a whirl. 'If that's right then Eddy and I are…are brothers. No wonder he thinks I look familiar. Perhaps I've got my father's eyes after all.

This is strange, it looks like my mother used her maiden name on my birth certificate. She must have decided to disown my father then…unless of course he never knew about me.

I must have been the new born baby when my father was having an affair with Eddy's step mother, Beverley, then. Sadly not quite the same father figure for me as for Eddy.

John studied the documents side by side and had difficulty believing what he was seeing.

'Next problem, how the hell do I break the news to Eddy? Will this send him over the top? Especially now.'

Chapter Eighty-two

Meanwhile two nurses from the hospital were on their way back from lunch when they spotted someone on the roof of the four storey Imagine Institute building. The man was standing precariously near the edge.

'Oh my God!' Kathryn said, putting her hand to her mouth.

'What is it?', her companion asked.

'Look Lyn. On the roof!' Kathryn pointed.

'Oh heavens! What's he doing up there? Do you think that he's going to jump?'

'Can you make out who it is?' Kathryn asked, shielding her eyes from the sun. 'Is it one of ours?'

'Yes. I think... I think it's Eddy,' Lyn replied nervously. 'I didn't think he was one of the vulnerable ones on the suicide watch list.'

'Well somethings' obviously upset him.

'Quick, we'd better tell someone.'

The women bounded in to reception and were relieved to see Laura at her desk..

'Quick Laura, there's someone on the roof who looks like they might jump.'

'Oh no! Do we know who it is?' Laura asked.

'Yes. We think that it's Eddy.'

'Oh no, not Eddy.' Laura repeated in shock, she quickly telephoned John's office.

John answered quickly, putting down the birth certificates he'd been re-reading.

'Hi Laura,' he answered.

'John, quick. Eddy is on the roof and it looks like he's going to jump,' she said in alarm.

'Oh no! Not now,' John blurted. 'OK leave it with me.'

John dashed out of his office, ran up the staircase and burst out on to the roof. Immediately he could see that it was Eddy.

He was standing right on the edge of the building. Cautiously John approached him walking slowly across the bitumen roof covering.

Eddy heard him approaching but continued to stare at the drop to the bottom of the building.

'Hello Eddy. I don't know about you but I get vertigo standing too close to big drops. Why don't you stand back from the edge and we can talk.'

'No. I've had enough,' he said, despondently. I can't cope with it anymore. It's all too much.'

'Damn, perhaps the trip to the crash site was a bridge too far,' John thought. 'Perhaps the Professor was right in his warning after all.'

'I'm sure we can sort this out without you having to take such drastic steps,' John suggested.

'Why? What's the point? I've nothing to live for. My girlfriend, Sheila has been lying to me. She isn't who she said she was. She's that television lady, the investigative reporter called Sophie Mcbid. She's been wearing a wig and false teeth.

'Oh it's that woman he's upset about, It's not the trip after all. Thank goodness for that' John thought, feeling relieved. 'I did warn you to be careful with her,' John reminded him unhelpfully.

'Yes, I know you did. But I loved her. Now Sheila has told me she never liked me in the first place.'

'I'm sorry, but it sounds like you've found out the hard way.'

'Yes she lied to me'. Eddy sobbed.

'What about Marilyn? Isn't she your real girlfriend? After all, you saved her life twice now, didn't you? So you must have loved her. And she is always defending you against other horrible people.'

'No, I ditched her for Sheila.'

'Oh Eddy, sorry to hear that.'

'I don't know who I am. You've made me remember horrors that I wanted to forget. Nobody will miss me,' Eddy said quietly, looking down at the people spectating at the bottom of the tall building.

'You have a lot to live for. You have friends. Lots of friends,' John said desperately trying to recall his suicide training. 'Keep them talking,' he seemed to remember.

'It's no good, I just can't think. My head… my head is full of… of ummm 'Cotton wool,' Eddy explained. It. It… it hurts to think.'

'Where exactly?' the doctor probed, trying to win more time.

'Here at the back of my head,' Eddy said touching his head. 'And in the front here, above my eyes.'

'Can you remember what that's called ?' John asked.

'No…it just hurts to think,' Eddy explained.

'Ok. I think we are talking about a headache, that's all. Nothing to worry about,' John suggested trying to lighten the conversation.

'It could be a tumour,' Eddy suggested pessimistically.

'No, not from your description,' John refuted his suggestion

'This is a waste of time,' Eddy said, swaying on the edge.

'Umm…You mentioned your girlfriend has given you up,' John said, desperately thinking of things to say. 'How did you get to know her?'

'Sheila was kind to me when the yobs attacked me.'

'Step away from the edge Eddy. You're making me nervous,' John said wiping his sweaty palms in his trousers.

Eddy did as John suggested but wobbled as he moved back a pace.

'Woah, steady on Eddy,' John said rushing towards him.

'I'm OK thanks,' Eddy replied and put his hand up to signal that he didn't want John to come any closer.

'Do you mean the woman who helped you after the protest march?'

'Yes.'

'You obviously realise she was using you?'

'I do now, Eddy said despondently.'

'She was using you to get to the Professor and me. I found her out too,' John revealed.

'But she didn't have to be angry with me though did she?' Eddy snivelled.

'I don't think she was interested in you in the first place. She set you up to pump you for information about the hospital. Yes, she was definitely using you,' John reiterated.

'She said she loved me,' Eddy wailed.'

'No. She was just trying to get a story to further her television career.'

'Then that's even worse. That's a horrible thing to do.' Eddy stepped closer to the edge again.

'Look, look Eddy at this, your photo,' John directed urgently, showing him a small photograph and holding it at arm's length towards him.

'I don't have any photos. It's not mine,' Eddy muttered soulfully.

'Look, step away from the edge and look. Just… just look here,' John implored.

Eddy wobbled as he stepped one step away from the edge, turned and looked at the photograph. 'Who is it ? That man looks…looks a bit. a bit like you.'

'Yes it does doesn't it?' John agreed.

'Oh this is making my head hurt,' Eddy said wobbling.'

'Steady… hold on please,' John said, reluctantly moving near to Eddy on the edge. 'I found this photo in your file.'

'No. It's not mine. I don't remember having any photos,' Eddy said, moving back towards the edge again.

'Yes you did,' John insisted. 'When you first started having…having treatment, they took all your possessions, including this photo, away from you. I gather they thought these were holding you back from well… getting over your depression and starting to get better. It was buried in your file.'

'What are you saying? I don't understand,' Eddy demanded..'

'I'm saying that I believe this photograph is of you and your family. That woman presumably is your step mother. That little boy is you and that man there is your father… And…he is my father too,' John revealed, feeling good about being able to speak about his own paternal link for the first time in his life.

Chapter Eighty-three

'Your father! How can he be your father too?' Eddy said sceptically. You're lying to me.'

'No I'm not,' John replied quickly.

'How do you know that?'

'Well I wanted to know more about you to be able to help you.'

'Yes, but what's that got to do with my father?'

'I sent for a copy of your birth certificate from England.'

'England?'

'Yes, and while I was at it, I sent for a copy of mine too. I have just received the documents today.'

'So, what did you discover?'

'Remember me telling you that I grew up without a father in my life. In other words I never knew who my father was because my mother wouldn't tell me anything about him.'

'Yes.'

'Well I...I found out today who he was. And, well that...that I am...I am your brother!'

Eddy turned at this revelation. 'What do you mean, my brother?' he demanded sceptically.

'Yes. You and I are brothers. Your father and my father was the same man. We have the same Mother too.'

'You're lying. How is that possible? How do you know? Eddy demanded'

'The birth certificates prove it. If you come off the roof I will show you.'

'Why should I believe you?'

'I'm as surprised as you. But I am also extremely delighted with the news,' John smiled.

Eddy came away from the edge and approached John. He took the photograph from him and studied the black and white image closely again.

'Wait, yes I think I remember it now,' he revealed. They took it away from me. And I hated them for doing that. I think I got a belting when I tried to get it back.'

'Oh yes; the *appropriate physical discipline*' entry in his notes, John recalled.

'The truth is, you and I were separated when we were infants. Our Dad brought you here to Australia and my, our Mum, stayed in England and changed her surname.

'I didn't know about you and you didn't know about me,' John beamed. 'Our mother had a baby picture hidden in her bedside cabinet and I spotted it one day. When I asked who the baby was, she said none of your business and told me off for interfering with her stuff. So it must have been you as a baby,' John revealed. 'I assume that you haven't been in touch with her?'

'No. I don't know anything about her,' Eddy revealed.

'Well I'm sure that Mother will be delighted that I have found you after all these years.' John added.

Eddy looked into John's smiling face and hugged him. 'My brother. My mother,' he sobbed. 'What is she like, my mother?' Eddy let the word 'mother' echo around his mind. 'Mother,' he repeated.

'OUR mother,' John emphasised the word our. 'She has white hair and an infectious laugh. She has a new partner and is very happy at last. I never knew the reason for her depression until now. I think it was because she had lost you in her life,' he suggested.

'Oh that's so sad,' Eddy croaked.

'Life has been so unfair for you Eddy,' John said sadly.

'What do you mean?'

'Because you were misdiagnosed when you were a child, you have missed out on a lot of life's experiences.'

Your obvious intellect was cruelly sedated over all those years and you have missed out on achieving your potential. You could have been a Doctor after all,' John reflected.

'So many of life's experiences have passed you by,' John continued, with a lump in his throat. 'But I will help you regain your quality of life. Your dignity Eddy.'

'Thank you brother,' Eddy said emotionally.

'I want to make up for it somehow,' John continued. 'To give you some joy and fun back in your life. But first we'll get you off those damn pills that the Professor has been giving you.'

'Thank you,' Eddy said filling up.

John studied the photograph again. 'So this is the father, that I never knew,' he thought. 'I tell you what, I'll even shave my beard off and really look like him,' John suggested. They laughed.

'Come on brother, let's go and make up for those lost years.' John suggested smiling.

The pair made their way off the roof with arms around each other's shoulders, passing a puzzled Laura who had come up to offer her assistance.

THE END

Chapter Eighty-four
Epilogue

Blood Brothers

Despite the revelation that they were 'blood' brothers, Eddy and John took some time to really bond. Having lived very different lives, switching off from the Doctor patient relationship took some time, especially for John.

Eddy took John on a poignant visit to his father's grave and they both laid flowers.

The pair now go fishing together, a new hobby for John.

Eddy

As Eddy's next of kin, John eventually persuaded the Professor to remove him from the drug trial and Eddy was slowly 'weaned off' all his medication.

As a result Eddy's mental state slowly improved. Plans are being made to move him from the sheltered housing to a new flat of his own.

Eddy and Marilyn are still good friends.

Our Mother

John rang his Mother to tell her about finding Eddy. Naturally she didn't believe it at first, but finally accepted that her toddler son had been found and had grown into a man.

John explained about Eddy's background so she was aware of Eddy's mannerisms.

Mum and partner have arranged to visit Manly soon.

John and Laura

John is still thoroughly enjoying his life 'down under' in New South Wales. In spite of having brother Eddy in his life, he is not allowing it to distract him from ticking off all the adventurous activities and experiences on his bucket list.

John and Laura continue their loving relationship but maintain their own accommodation to keep their personal space.

Marilyn

Following a course of hypnotherapy, John has found the cause of Marilyn's aggression and has 'talked' her out of her anger issues caused by being ignored by her parents.

The fire episode that she talks about is believed to have been caused by an electrical fire that Marilyn had nothing to do with, but she blamed herself after saying that she hated her brother and sister.

The Professor

The Professor accepted John's apology for his out of character outburst when he accused the academic of professional 'skulduggery'.

He is still looking for the golden bullet that will 'cure' ALL mental illness and has started working with the complexities of the link between mental health and DNA.

The drug company are still supporting the Professors work. The funding is going into the correct Institute account as it always did.

Sophie Mcbid

Sophie Mcbid was found guilty of manslaughter but cleared of murder after convincing the jury that Digger Lucas had attacked her first.

She was nevertheless sent to prison with a four year sentence.

Although Sophie lost her career outside. Behind bars, the women's prison service made use of her talents in getting her to run their own 'in house' entertainment centre.

However, her past caught up with her. She was physically attacked by some inmates whom she had got imprisoned when she exposed their criminal activities, during the making of her documentaries.

The producer and graphic designer were subjected to a professional misconduct enquiry about other programmes that Sophie Mcbid had fronted. They were castigated for their collusion and allowing misinformation to be broadcast.

Also by the Same Author

Godsons – Counting Sunsets

Godsons – Counting Sunsets is a heartening story, charting the stubbornness of the human spirit to let the precious gift of life slip away without a fight to the bitter end.

Multimillionaire Geoffery Foster has been diagnosed with terminal cancer and has irrationally swapped his luxurious Monaco penthouse for a single room in a Cotswolds hospice in Gloucestershire England.

Determined to maximise his remaining days and impressed by the selfless humanity shown by his hospice nurse, Andy Spider, Geoffery decides to redress his neglected Godfather responsibilities.

Together Andy and Geoffery embark on a journey to track down and improve the lot of Geoffery's three Godsons.

But will resolving the problems of childhood Meningitis amputee Tim, the alcoholic 'drop out' James and the abused husband Rupert, be too much for Geoffery's frail health.

Added to his challenges, a drunken and intimate wedding reception encounter with a former girlfriend comes back to haunt Geoffery as he also gambles with his life in the hands of a woman spurned.

Counting Sunsets becomes the abacus on which Geoffery records his remaining days.

Proving, *'It's never too late to be who you could have been,'* George Elliot.

The Godsons Legacy

Andy Spider continues to be the glue that cements the three Godsons together as they expectantly await the release of their legacy from Geoffery Foster's will.

But surely even this pillar of society will be distracted from his task when tempted by the radiant beauty of Nadine.

Mesmerised by the exotic Monaco nightlife, his stoic resolve is weakened by lack of sleep and too much alcohol.

Pallbearers wearing Basques, Murder, Blackmail, Fear, Lust, a Motorway Crash, a runaway teenager, and police Investigations are the unexpected consequences of Geoffery's legacy as he still controls their lives FROM BEYOND THE GRAVE.

The story is set in Gloucestershire England, near the beautiful Cotswold Hills.

The Godsons Inheritance

The three Godsons have to work harmoniously to place the final piece in the inheritance puzzle for the release of their legacy.

But the wayward Tim makes it a challenging exercise. His self-centred, bloody-minded arrogance means the whole intricate web of relationships is jeopardised. Will his heart bring him back in line or will he still be ruled by his head?

Meanwhile Rupert is continually in fear of his vicious megalomaniacal wife and James is clinging on to life desperate for a liver transplant.

Young army veteran Carrie is haunted by the trauma of active service.

Ben a young carer for his alcoholic Mother inadvertently opens up old wounds by looking for his father. Can fellow young carer Janie help or hinder Ben's traumatic life?

Andy is having a bad time in his personal life, haunted by a late night indiscretion, and frustrated by having to coordinate the activities of the three Godsons.

The story comes to a dramatic and exciting conclusion but is it the end. In this the third book in the Godsons series?

Godsons – That Woman

It all started so well with the lovely Christening in the ancient church, but then things started going downhill.

Someone was spying on the christening party as they left the church.

Then it got worse. A disputed will has triggered kidnap, arson, and murder.

Who's behind the blood lust? Surely the chief suspect is dead?

Ben carrying a knife is strictly a no-no, so how does it become a life saver?

Can Nadine survive her nightmare visit to the UK challenging Geoffery Foster's will?

An overstretched police force is being led a merry dance as suspicions fall on 'THAT WOMAN'

Unexploded Love

A love triangle is already an explosive situation without the added complication of an unexploded bomb.

But the Luftwaffe's 1944 legacy of a large bomb exposes a burgeoning romance and throws together the three people in the love match.

Trapped in a collapsed hole with a ticking WW2 bomb for company, the love cheat's hope of escape is in the hands of the man he is cuckolding.

Will the frantic race against time succeed? Or will the husband take revenge?

The stark outcome can only be a blast from the past or UNEXPLODED LOVE?.

Gurney Leafmould - The Pied Piper of Calamity

With great DIY aspirations, there is nothing Gurney Leafmould won't tackle – but intent and results are poles apart.

For 'Do it Yourself' means upheaval when Gurney is holding the tools
 This is a lively and humorous tale of DIY disasters created by Gurney, a hapless DIYer.

His calamitous CV includes house demolition and fire; a car blaze and a farm inferno coupled together with failed car maintenance and hospital chaos, which are all neatly wrapped in EU red tape. Not to mention a very delicate DIY surgical transplant.
 Many wives and partners will recognise some of Gurney's 'attributes' in their own DIY champions.

Willing but incapable, he is a first class prat to his Mother-in-Law but to his long suffering wife, Gurney Leafmould is 'The Pied Piper of Calamity'.

Contains 'Adult Humour'

Gurney Leafmould - The Ministry of Disruption

Gurney Leafmould was a hapless DIYer but is now legally restrained by an ASBO preventing him from undertaking any more DIY projects.

Unable to pursue his real passion, he turns to Journalism and proves he is good at it.

However, his decision to become an investigative Journalist has disastrous consequences when he stumbles on to a state secret, an organisation called the Ministry Of Disruption (MOD).

By subsequently joining this 'clandestine organisation', Gurney hopes to 'blow the whistle' on their activities and get a major news scoop.

He discovers that the MOD, which was created during WW2 as a guerrilla force to disrupt invading forces; is still active today and conducting disruptive training exercises.

So, if you've been held up in a traffic jam; been stuck at an airport, delayed on a rail journey, the cause of which you could never find out...then it's likely you have been an unwitting 'casualty' of a MOD exercise.

This is the second humorous Gurney Leafmould novel.

AFGHAN BOY – The Impossible Dream

Mohammed (14) has been orphaned in a suicide bombing and rescued from underneath the debris of his destroyed family home by a British Soldier and his search dog,

However, the Soldier, the only person that seems to care for him, leaves shortly after the rescue, at the end of his posting.

But undeterred the boy travels half way around the world to find the soldier in the hope he would adopt him.

The journey is fraught with danger, and the boy confronts the many gruelling challenges; walking thousands of miles, often through sandstorms, braving armed gangs and in overloaded trucks, as well as a sinking dinghy, and the menacing refugee camp in Calais.

His many attempts to cross the channel are frustrated by the Border force.

Can he beat the odds of getting to the UK and then, if he does, of finding the soldier. Will being a Scout help him?

This is Mo's story, his 'IMPOSSIBLE DREAM'.

Vigilante Nurse

Rebecca Roberts, former army medic is usually unflappable, whether on a Middle East battlefield or the lawless streets of her hometown.

That was until she became unwittingly complicit in the death of her fiancé, Tony.
Guilt ridden by his loss she left the army and joined the NHS on the 'frontline' as an A & E nurse.

Respected for her cool head under pressure Rebecca takes the law into her own hands when she discovers her colleague, Amber, is being brutalised by her policeman husband.

Frustrated by police inaction, she metes out her own punishment to the abuser.

But the punishment goes wrong and she is pursued by an eagle eyed Detective Constable determined to get justice for his partner.

Nevertheless, Rebecca is undaunted; the adrenaline junkie gets her next high tackling major criminality including the drug gangs.

Despite her tough exterior she has a tender spot for the young and vulnerable and eventually even allows some romance to return to her life.

Tackling sex, drugs and violence, Rebecca is THE Vigilante Nurse.

CPSIA information can be obtained
at www.ICGtesting.com
Printed in the USA
LVHW012046120322
713318LV00001B/9